D1543901

Pediatric Cardiology and Cardiosurgery

Modern Problems in Paediatrics

Vol. 22

Series Editors
F. Falkner; N. Kretchmer, Berkeley, Calif.;
E. Rossi, Bern

Secretary General
H. Berger, Innsbruck

S. Karger · Basel · München · Paris · London · New York · Sydney

Pediatric Cardiology and Cardiosurgery

Volume Editors
G. Piero Belloli, Vicenza; *U. Squarcia*, Parma

73 figures and 65 tables, 1983

S. Karger · Basel · München · Paris · London · New York · Sydney

WS
290
I59
1981

Modern Problems in Paediatrics

LIBRARY
CORNELL UNIVERSITY
MEDICAL COLLEGE
NEW YORK CITY

OCT 1 7 1983

Drug Dosage

The authors and the publisher have exerted every effort to ensure that drug selection and dosage set forth in this text are in accord with current recommendations and practice at the time of publication. However, in view of ongoing research, changes in government regulations, and the constant flow of information relating to drug therapy and drug reactions, the reader is urged to check the package insert for each drug for any change in indications and dosage and for added warnings and precautions. This is particularly important when the recommended agent is a new and/or infrequently employed drug.

All right reserved

No part of this publication may be translated into other languages, reproduced or utilized in any form or by any means, electronic or mechanical, including photocopying, recording, microcopying, or by any information storage and retrieval system, without permission in writing from the publisher.

© Copyright 1983 by S.Karger AG, P.O. Box, CH–4009 Basel (Switzerland)
Printed in Switzerland by Benziger AG, Graphischer Betrieb, Einsiedeln
ISBN 3–8055–3593–7

Contents

Preface

Pediatric Cardiology and Cardiac Surgery are two relatively young spe-
cialities among pediatric disciplines, which have, however, constantly progressed at an amazingly fast pace. At the beginning of the 40s a Boston
pediatrician, Dr. *Hubbard*, diagnosed a patent ductus arteriosus and a pediatric surgeon, Dr. *Gross*, successfully performed the first surgical ligation of a
ductus. A few years later, in Baltimore, a pediatric cardiologist, Dr. *Helen
Taussig*, conceived the idea of creating a 'patent ductus' in children with
cyanosis from deficient pulmonary blood flow, and Dr. *Alfred Blalock*, a
vascular surgeon, successfully managed to suture a subclavian artery end-to-
side to a pulmonary artery, thus creating the Blalock-Taussig anastomosis.

From the combined work of cardiologists and cardiac surgeons a new
era began which would have brought to the most extraordinary results in
terms of survival and rehabilitation. Today, with the immense technical and
diagnostic means of modern medicine available, we can set our goals for
children with congenital heart disease not only in terms of survival but of
improved quality of life. Almost one percent of babies are born with congenital cardiac anomalies and in at least half of them the related problems arise in
the first year of life. For this reason progressively more and more attention
has focused on the challenges presented by the neonate with congenital heart
disease, and it is in this group that diagnosis and treatment is most reward-
ing.

The purpose of this volume is to highlight the recent advances in the
knowledge of the peculiar problems of the newborn and in the evaluation and
management of infants with heart disease. The first part of the volume deals
with general problems of the neonate with severe heart defects, and the
physiopathology of the ductus closure. The medical treatment of ductus

arteriosus has offered new possibilities to the pediatric cardiologist either
when closure of a patent ductus is required (as in a premature with respiratory distress syndrome), or when its patency is to be maintained to assure
pulmonary blood flow (as in pulmonary atresia), or systemic flow (as in
interrupted aortic arch). The immense technical resources of contemporary
medicine permit a remarkably precise anatomic and physiologic diagnosis of
the cardiovascular anomalies. Subsequent chapters of the volume are devoted to new methods of investigation, such as echo cardiography and nuclear
medicine. This part includes the presentation of the dynamic spatial recon-
structer, a prototype machine developed at the Mayo Clinic and being used
to achieve three-dimensional imaging of heart and vessels. Clinical and in-
strumental evaluation as well as early and late results of surgical correction
or palliation of specific cardiac conditions are presented. Coarctation of
aorta, tetralogy of Fallot, tricupid atresia, pulmonary atresia, transposition
of great vessels, truncus arteriosus, A-V canal, are the lesions presented and
discussed by different groups of experts in the clinical or surgical field.

The final chapters are devoted to the intraoperative technique of an-
esthesiological assistance and myocardial protection and to postoperative
monitoring of different parameters of pediatric cardiac patients. Both these
aspects have had profound impact on the final results of cardiac surgery.

The volume is made up by the contribution of some of the most outstanding groups of experts in the field of pediatric cardiology and cardiac
surgery working in Europe and North America. 'One of the great satisfac-
tions of medicine is being able to help those in need', Dr. *Helen Taussig* has
written with the wisdom of a person who dedicated her entire life to medicine.
It is great satisfaction of all of us, Scientific Editors and Co-Authors, having
tried to help those in need, now to offer our experience and knowledge to
others. Our final goal remains ultimately to improve the lives of children,
and to bring happiness to them and their families.

G. Piero Belloli
Umberto Squarcia

Mod. Probl. Paediat., vol. 22, pp. 1–6 (Karger, Basel 1983)

General Problems of Severe Heart Disease in the Newborn

Abraham M. Rudolph

Departments of Pediatrics, Obstetrics, Gynecology, and Reproductive Sciences, and Physiology, and Cardiovascular Research Institute, University of California, San Francisco, Calif., USA

Many congenital cardiac lesions are compatible with normal intrauterine survival and development, due to the presence of fetal vascular shunts, and the fact that blood is oxygenated in the placenta. After birth, when the function of gas exchange is taken over by the lungs, it is necessary to establish not only effective ventilation, but also an adequate pulmonary blood flow. Associated with elimination of the umbilical-placental circulation and establishment of the pulmonary circulation, the shunts through the ductus venosus, foramen ovale, and ductus arteriosus are curtailed within a few hours after birth, and the normal postnatal course of the circulation is achieved. In the presence of various congenital heart lesions, however, the fetal vascular shunts may delay onset of symptoms after birth, and may in fact permit survival of the infant. Closure of the shunt may result in rapid deterioration.

The symptomatology associated with congenital heart disease in the neonate may be considered on the basis of several pathophysiologic mechanisms. These include: Inadequate pulmonary blood flow: actual reduction in flow; decreased effective blood flow. Inadequate systemic blood flow. Left ventricular outflow obstruction. Pulmonary venous obstruction. Volume overloads: valvar insufficiency; shunts.

These may exist separately or be combined. It is apparent that in many congenital heart lesions the primary pathophysiology is not related to myocardial insufficiency, which is the most frequent concern in adults, but rather to disturbances in oxygen supply to the tissues. I will consider some of the factors influencing oxygen requirements and supply in the newborn infant, with particular reference to congenital heart disease.

Oxygen uptake in the lungs is determined by ventilation and pulmonary blood flow. If it is assumed that ventilation is normal, and diffusion of oxygen is normal, then oxygen uptake is directly related to the pulmonary blood flow, and to the oxygen-carrying capacity of the blood. Oxygen-carrying capacity is calculated from hemoglobin concentration (g/dl) $\times$ 1.34, and is expressed as ml/dl; it indicates the maximal amount of oxygen that can be taken up by hemoglobin. In addition, a small amount of oxygen is present in solution in blood. In congenital heart lesions in which pulmonary blood flow is reduced, as in pulmonary atresia, there is invariably a right-to-left shunt present, either through the foramen ovale or a ventricular septal defect; if this were not present, systemic blood flow could not be maintained and survival would not be possible. Contrary to general opinion, however, it is not the magnitude of the right-to-left shunt that determines the degree of cyanosis and the adequacy of oxygenation, but the actual pulmonary blood flow. The importance of hemoglobin concentration cannot be overemphasized, because the amount of oxygen that can be taken up in the lungs is directly related to it. There is a limit to this beneficial effect because when hemoglobin concentration is increased markedly the associated rise of hematocrit may increase the blood viscosity sufficiently to interfere with tissue perfusion. This is not very important until hematocrit levels exceed about 68–70%.

In aortopulmonary transposition, pulmonary blood flow may be normal or high, and yet severe hypoxemia may occur. In this condition, it is effective pulmonary blood flow that determines the degree of oxygenation; this is directly related to the magnitude of the bidirectional shunt. The right-to-left and left-to-right shunts must be equal, or else in a short period of time, either the pulmonary or systemic blood volume would be depleted. The effective pulmonary blood flow represents the volume of systemic venous blood that reaches the lungs for oxygenation and then returns to the systemic arterial circulation, this is directly related to the magnitude of the shunts.

When actual or effective pulmonary blood flow is markedly reduced, in association with the right-to-left shunt there is a decrease in systemic arterial oxygen saturation (hypoxemia) and a reduced delivery of oxygen to the tissues. In order to obtain adequate oxygen for metabolic needs extraction is increased, but when the limits to this compensation are reached, inadequate oxygen supply or hypoxia develops. This results in an increase in anaerobic metabolism, with increased lactic acid formation, and the development of acidemia. Because lactic acid does not undergo its final metabolism to carbon dioxide and water, CO_2 production is reduced and arterial PCO_2 levels usually do not increase. The lack of increase in PCO_2 is partly related to the increased elimination of CO_2 in the lungs associated with hyperventilation.

The amount of oxygen delivered to the tissues by the systemic circulation is determined by the systemic blood flow and the oxygen content of blood; the latter is determined by oxygen saturation of hemoglobin and the oxygen capacity, or hemoglobin concentration. Thus, reduced oxygen delivery may occur when oxygen saturation is reduced, as mentioned above, in cyanotic heart disease, or if systemic blood flow or hemoglobin concentrations are decreased.

Systemic blood flow to the whole body is reduced when cardiac output is restricted, as with severe aortic stenosis or aortic atresia with hypoplastic left heart. Blood flow to the lower body is decreased in infants with aortic arch interruption or aortic coarctation. The importance of the ductus arteriosus in determining systemic blood flow in these conditions is discussed in the section on the ductus arteriosus (pp. 7–14). The ultimate physiological and biochemical consequences of reduced systemic blood flow do not differ from those of decreased pulmonary blood flow. Even though arterial oxygen saturation may be normal, with severe reduction of systemic blood flow there will be an inadequate oxygen supply to the tissues, with the development of anaerobic metabolism culminating in severe metabolic acidemia.

The actual oxygen uptake in the tissues is determined by the quantity being delivered and the extraction of oxygen. Thus, within limits, the extraction can be increased, and venous PO_2 and oxygen saturation are reduced. The type of hemoglobin is most important in determining the amount of oxygen that can be extracted from blood in tissues. As can be seen in figure 1, the oxygen equilibration curve of blood in which the hemoglobin is of fetal type is shifted to the left of that of blood with adult type hemoglobin. When arterial PO_2 is in the high range (i.e., above about 70 mm Hg) and venous PO_2 at the usual level of about 35–40 mm Hg, blood with adult type hemoglobin will release much more oxygen than fetal blood. The importance of this is that a greater blood flow is required to deliver the same amount of oxygen to the tissues. Therefore, a reduction of systemic blood flow has a more serious effect in the newborn period, when most hemoglobin is of the fetal type. Fetal hemoglobin as a percentage of total hemoglobin rapidly falls to near zero by 8–10 weeks after birth.

Left ventricular outflow obstruction occurs in the immediate newborn period with aortic atresia and critical aortic stenosis, and within a few days or weeks in infants with severe aortic coarctation. These conditions are associated with reduced systemic blood flow and frequently left ventricular failure. The importance of the ductus arteriosus in maintaining systemic blood flow is discussed in the section on the ductus. Left ventricular

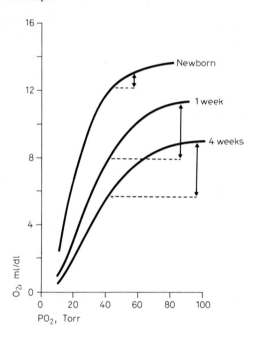

Fig. 1. The effects of type of hemoglobin and oxygen dissociation curve on oxygen release at the tissue site are shown. In the immediate newborn period, hemoglobin concentration is high; therefore, oxygen content at full saturation (oxygen capacity) is also high. With the fall in hemoglobin concentration in the first few weeks after birth, oxygen capacity is reduced. In the newborn period, when most hemoglobin is of the fetal type, the amount of oxygen released from arterial PO_2 levels to venous PO_2 levels is quite low. With replacement of fetal by adult hemoglobin, the amount of oxygen released from each volume of blood is greater, even though oxygen capacity is less.

failure is a consequence of the increased afterload on the left ventricle, which results in an increase in systolic pressure, in end-diastolic pressure, with left atrial and pulmonary venous pressure elevation. If the foramen ovale is incompetent or an atrial septal defect is present, the left atrial pressure may not increase as dramatically as when foramen ovale closure is effective because an atrial left-to-right shunt will occur. The increase in left atrial and pulmonary venous pressures, if marked, will cause pulmonary edema with respiratory distress. Pulmonary edema interferes with gas exchange in the lungs and blood PCO_2 may increase and PO_2 fall.

Pulmonary edema in congenital heart disease may result from mechanisms other than left ventricular failure. Obstructions between the lung and the left ventricle may not present any difficulty in the fetus because pulmonary blood flow is low. However, when pulmonary blood flow increases after birth, an obstruction, which may not have been of consequence when flow was low, may then become severe. This phenomenon may result from mitral stenosis or atresia with a small foramen ovale, or from cor triatriatum, but the commonest cause is total anomalous pulmonary venous connection with obstruction. When pulmonary venous drainage is infradiaphragmatic, if the veins enter a portal vein, the ductus venosus may be important in determining onset of symptoms. While open, obstruction may not be severe, but with closure serious obstruction may develop. The ductus arteriosus also influences the clinical features and onset of symptoms. When pulmonary venous obstruction supervenes, if the ductus arteriosus is open, pulmonary arterial pressure cannot exceed systemic arterial pressure, pulmonary blood flow tends to be limited, and, because the volume of blood in the lungs is not greatly increased, pulmonary edema may not be severe. However, due to the restriction of pulmonary blood flow, cyanosis may be marked. When the ductus closes, pulmonary arterial pressure can increase above systemic levels and the pulmonary blood flow will increase, causing a further increase in pulmonary venous pressure and pulmonary edema.

Volume overload of the left or right sides of the heart is common in congenital cardiac lesions. With the common defects, such as atrial, ventricular, or aortopulmonary communications, there is usually no problem during the early neonatal period because the shunts only become large as pulmonary vascular resistance falls. Lesions that produce volume overload in the newborn period would usually have caused difficulties in utero and the baby may be born in cardiac failure. This group of conditions includes mitral, tricuspid, pulmonary, or aortic insufficiency or aortic-left ventricular tunnel. Shunts that may cause volume overload with cardiac failure in the newborn period are usually arteriovenous fistulae, particularly large cerebral arteriovenous fistulae.

In general, the therapeutic approach to infants with cardiorespiratory distress has been to administer oxygen to attempt to increase oxygen delivery. In cases of reduced cardiac output, digitalis, usually as digoxin, is administered in an attempt to provide more blood flow to the tissues. Also, diuretics are given to attempt to reduce pulmonary edema. In most instances, surgical therapy is required on an urgent basis.

I would like to recommend that medical management be approached with considerations of oxygen supply and oxygen requirements. Oxygen supply to the body in infants with reduced actual or effective pulmonary blood flow can be increased to some extent by administering 100% oxygen.

However, the amount of oxygen that can be added is limited. Because pulmonary venous blood hemoglobin is fully saturated, the only additional amount of oxygen that can be provided is that dissolved in blood; this is a relatively small amount and may be of little consequence. As mentioned in the section on ductus arteriosus, pulmonary blood flow may be increased with prostaglandin E_1. Another important means by which oxygen uptake can be increased is by raising hemoglobin level by blood transfusion.

Systemic oxygen supply may be increased by prostaglandin E_1 in those infants in whom systemic blood flow is ductus dependent.

Cardiac output is not usually greatly improved by digoxin administration in the immediate neonatal period, especially in premature infants, but catecholamine infusions may be more effective. One possible means of improving tissue oxygen supply in the presence of reduced systemic blood flow is to exchange fetal hemoglobin with adult blood. This could increase the oxygen delivery at the tissue level. This approach has not been used extensively.

Equally important to increasing oxygen supply is to attempt to reduce oxygen requirements. Because oxygen consumption is greatly increased by exposure to cold, which increases metabolic activity, it is important to maintain these infants with cardiorespiratory distress in a neutral thermal environment. The oxygen requirements could also be reduced by sedation to lessen body activity and anxiety. Morphine is very effective for this purpose, but one should be prepared to provide respiratory assistance if respirations are depressed. Tracheal intubation with assisted respiration, and use of muscle relaxants may considerably reduce oxygen requirements by eliminating the work of breathing and also by restricting muscular activity. Finally, general anesthesia may be used for short periods, prior to planned surgery, to reduce metabolism to a basal level and thus limit body needs for oxygen.

Abraham M. Rudolph, MD, Department of Pediatrics, Obstetrics, Gynecology, and Reproductive Sciences, and Physiology, and Cardiovascular Research Institute, University of California, San Francisco, CA 94143 (USA)

Mod. Probl. Paediat., vol. 22, pp. 7–14 (Karger, Basel 1983)

The Ductus arteriosus: Physiological and Therapeutic Considerations

Abraham M. Rudolph

Departments of Pediatrics, Obstetrics, Gynecology, and Reproductive Sciences, and Physiology, and Cardiovascular Research Institute, University of California, San Francisco, Calif., USA

The ductus arteriosus connects the pulmonary trunk with the descending aorta. Prenatally, it is important in blood distribution and in reducing cardiac work. Postnatal closure usually occurs rapidly; if this does not occur, symptoms of cardiac failure may develop. However, in certain congenital heart lesions, ductus closure may initiate the onset of clinical manifestations.

During fetal life, blood is oxygenated in the placenta and returns to the fetal body via the umbilical vein. The oxygenated blood mixes with systemic venous blood in the inferior vena cava. Recently we have shown, however, that umbilical venous blood bypassing the liver through the ductus venosus, is preferentially distributed through the foramen ovale, to enter the left atrium, left ventricle and ascending aorta [1]. Distal inferior vena caval blood is preferentially directed across the tricuspid valve. Almost the total superior vena caval return passes through the tricuspid valve to the right ventricle. Right ventricular blood thus has a lower oxygen saturation than that in the left ventricle, and pulmonary arterial oxygen saturation is lower than that in the ascending aorta. The right ventricle ejects about 65 % of total fetal cardiac output and, because pulmonary vascular resistance is very high in the fetus, most of the output of the right ventricle passes through the ductus arteriosus to the descending aorta [2]. About 85 % of right ventricular blood, or about 60 % of the total cardiac output, passes through the ductus arteriosus. It is thus apparent that the ductus arteriosus serves two important functions during fetal life. First, because the blood of lower oxygen saturation in the right ventricle is directed through the ductus to the descending aorta, venous blood is preferentially directed to the umbilical-placental circulation where gas exchange occurs; thus, the ductus facilitates oxygen uptake by the fetus. The second function of the ductus is to reduce the total work load on the fetal heart. If the ductus was not present, all right ventricular blood would be ejected through the pulmonary trunk to the pulmonary circulation; this blood would return to the left atrium and then be ejected by the left ventricle. It would thus be necessary for the left ventricle to eject a large volume, both for supplying the fetal body, as well as for the placenta. In providing the bypass of the lungs, the ductus greatly reduces the volume load on the heart.

Following birth, the ductus arteriosus closes rapidly; in different species functional closure is accomplished in minutes to several hours. Initial closure is the result of smooth muscle constriction, and permanent closure by fibrosis follows. The actual mechanisms responsible for ductus arteriosus closure have not been fully delineated. However, it is well known that an increase in the oxygen tension to which the ductus is exposed, usually results in constriction; the less mature the animal or infant, the less sensitive is the ductus to oxygen. Recently, it has become apparent that prostaglandins are important in regulating the ductus arteriosus both before and after birth. Administration of inhibitors of prostaglandin synthesis to maternal rats results in early constriction of the ductus in the fetuses after birth [3], and in sheep, prostaglandin synthesis inhibitors cause constriction of the ductus arteriosus in utero [4]. This ductus constriction can be overcome by infusing PGE_1.

Prostaglandin synthesis inhibitors block production of all prostaglandins, and the actual prostaglandin responsible for maintaining ductus patency in the fetus has not yet been defined. Ductus arteriosus rings incubated in tissue baths release large quantities of prostacyclin (PGI_2) and smaller amounts of prostaglandin E_2 (PGE_2) [5]. However, testing the sensitivity of the ductus to various prostaglandins, shows that PGE_2 is considerably more potent in causing dilatation of the ductus than is either PGI_2 or $PGF_2\alpha$ [6]. In adults, circulating concentrations of prostaglandins are very low, but in fetal lambs, PGE_2 and $PGF_2\alpha$ concentrations are considerably greater; these concentrations fall to adult levels within a few hours after birth [7]. The hypothesis has therefore been considered that the ductus arteriosus is kept open by circulating PGE_2 in the fetus, and that after birth, constriction results from both a reduction in circulating prostaglandin concentrations and the increase in arterial oxygen tension which normally occurs.

Studies with isolated lamb ductus rings have shown that the immature ductus, which constricts less with oxygen, is more sensitive to the effects of prostaglandin synthesis inhibitors than the mature ductus [8]. Thus, if the ductus is maximally constricted with both oxygen and indomethacin, a larger percentage of constriction is produced by inhibition of prostaglandin synthesis in immature animals and a greater percentage by oxygen, in mature animals. The ductus arteriosus thus progressively loses its sensitivity to PGE_2 with increasing maturity.

The Ductus arteriosus in Congenital Heart Disease
Ductus-Dependent Pulmonary Blood Flow

Oxygenation of the infant after birth is achieved by establishing ventilation and adequate pulmonary blood flow. In congenital heart lesions with right ventricular outflow obstruction, or with tricuspid atresia, systemic venous blood may not be able to reach the lungs for oxygenation, unless shunts are present. In the newborn infant with pulmonary atresia, the only route by which blood can reach the lungs is through the ductus arteriosus. With tricuspid atresia, in the absence of a ventricular septal defect, patency of the ductus arteriosus also is essential for providing blood flow to the lungs. In the early postnatal period, when the ductus is still open, an adequate pulmonary blood flow is maintained, and although cyanosis may be evident, it is not severe, and oxygen uptake may be adequate for body needs. As the ductus begins to constrict, pulmonary blood flow is decreased, cyanosis increases, and increasing hypoxemia develops; when oxygen supply falls markedly, anaerobic metabolism increases, with progressive metabolic acidemia. The surgical management of these infants has been either to create some form of aortopulmonary shunt, or, if possible, to open the right ventricular outflow.

PGE$_1$ has been administered to these infants prior to surgery, in attempts to dilate the ductus, improve pulmonary blood flow, and increase oxygen uptake. This has been very effective in the majority of infants, resulting in a rapid increase of arterial blood PO_2 levels within minutes, and, when metabolic acidemia has been present, it has improved gradually. Usually the increase in PO_2 has been most dramatic in those infants with the lowest arterial PO_2 level [9]. PO_2 usually has increased to about 40–45 Torr; if PO_2 has been at this level, there has not been any further significant rise. PGE$_1$ is rapidly metabolized in the body and therefore it must be given by continuous intravascular infusion, either through an umbilical arterial catheter advanced to the descending aorta adjacent to the ductus, or intravenously. It is given at an initial rate of 0.1 μg/kg b.w./min, but as soon as improvement in PO$_2$ is noted, the infusion rate can be reduced to 0.05 μg/kg/min, and it may even be reduced further to 0.025 μg/kg/min. Usually the infusion has been given for a few hours until the infant's oxygenation and metabolic status have improved and surgery has been performed. However, the intravenous infusion has been continued for as long as 2–3 months in some cases, particularly premature infants, in whom surgical shunt procedures may be technically difficult to accomplish. No evidence of diminishing response has been noted in long-term infusions.

PGE$_2$ has been administered orally in a group of infants, for periods of 4–6 months [10]. Although this has been effective in maintaining ductus patency, it produces diarrhea, often of severe degree. However, it has been suggested that if the administration of the prostaglandin is continued, the diarrhea tends to improve.

Ductus-Dependent Systemic Flow

Postnatally, if the ductus arteriosus remains patent, blood usually flows from the aorta to the pulmonary artery, in association with the decrease in pulmonary, and increase in systemic, vascular resistances. In certain congenital heart lesions, blood flows from the pulmonary artery to the aorta through the ductus, which now becomes crucial in maintaining systemic blood flow. This occurs in lesions such as aortic atresia or severe aortic stenosis. In infants with interruption of the aortic arch, the only means by which blood can reach the descending aorta is through the ductus. If the ductus arteriosus constricts, blood flow to the descending aorta and lower body pressure falls. This interferes with tissue perfusion, resulting in oliguria or anuria and in tissue hypoxia with progressive metabolic acidemia.

Infusion of PGE$_1$ in infants with aortic arch interruption has resulted in dilatation of the ductus with an increase in the descending aortic pressure, improved perfusion of the lower body, and gradual resolution of the metabolic acidemia [11]. The drug is infused at the same rate outlined above for cyanotic infants. However, the results are not uniformly as good as in the cyanotic group, for no obvious reason. It is apparent that the later after birth that the infusion is initiated, the less likely it is to be effective. This conforms to the observations made in isolated lamb ductus, in which there is a decrease in response to prostaglandin with increasing maturity. When it is effective, PGE$_1$ has been useful in improving metabolic and urinary status in infants prior to surgery.

Many infants with juxtaductal aortic coarctation do not have any evidence of aortic obstruction at birth, but develop evidence of stenosis after several days or weeks. One theory proposed to explain the postnatal development of aortic coarctation is that the smooth muscle of the ductus arteriosus extends to the aortic wall, and that when the ductus constricts, aortic constriction develops. We have proposed another mechanism that can explain development of aortic coarctation some time after birth in association with ductus constriction [12]. In most infants with juxtaductal coarctation, a posterolateral shelf projects into the aorta opposite the ductus. During fetal life, and while the aortic end of the ductus is patent after birth, there is an adequate passage around the shelf from either the pulmonary trunk or the ascending aorta, to the descending aorta. However, when the ductus constricts, aortic obstruction develops and pressure in the descending aorta falls; if severe enough, tissue perfusion to the lower body will be inadequate. Also the acute obstruction increases ascending aortic and left ventricular pressure, and may result in acute left ventricular failure.

Infusion of PGE_1 has produced dramatic improvement in many of these infants, with increase in descending aortic and reduction in ascending aortic and left ventricular pressures. In some instances, the systolic pressure difference has disappeared. Associated with this, left ventricular end-diastolic pressure also falls and all clinical evidences of cardiac failure may disappear. The effectiveness of prostaglandin appears to be related to age after birth; the younger the infant, the more likely is PGE_1 to improve the infant's condition.

Side Effects of PGE_1

Infusion of PGE_1 is associated with a number of side effects, most of which are of little consequence, but several may be life threatening. In a recent review [13], these occurred in about 40% of patients. The more important effects were hypotension in about 20%, apnea or respiratory depression in 12%, and pyrexia and tremulousness in 16%. In many instances of pyrexia and tremulousness, the symptoms disappear if infusion is continued. Hypotension is not usually serious, and if the rate of infusion is reduced, the effect on the ductus will be maintained, but blood pressure usually recovers. The most important concern is the possible development of apnea; therefore, in any infant to whom PGE_1 is administered, there should be the facilities and skills for tracheal intubation and ventilation.

It has been suggested that PGE_1 infusions may damage the wall of the ductus when used for several days [14]. This is based on histological study of the ductus on infants at autopsy, but no clinical evidence of any subsequent difficulty has yet been encountered. It has also been noted that changes in the small blood vessels in the lung may occur [15], but no apparent difficulty relating to these changes has been encountered. It is possible that late effects may result from long-term infusions. Cortical hypertrophy of long bones has been noted in some infants after prolonged infusions, but the bones have gradually returned to normal.

Persistent Patency of the Ductus arteriosus in Premature Infants

Although the ductus arteriosus closes within a few hours after birth in mature infants, closure is frequently delayed for days or even weeks in premature infants; the lower the gestational age, the higher the incidence of persistent patency of the ductus. The exact mechanisms responsible for the delayed ductus closure are not known, but, as mentioned above, it could be explained by the lesser sensitivity to oxygen constriction, and the greater sensitivity to relaxation by prostaglandin, of the immature ductus. Many infants do not develop symptoms relating to the ductus, but if the left-to-right shunt is large, evidences of cardiac failure may occur and, also, because diastolic pressure may be very low, tissue perfusion may be interfered with. Also, particularly in premature infants with associated hyaline membrane disease, persistent patency of the ductus may aggravate the respiratory distress and interfere with ventilation so that arterial blood PCO_2 rises and ventilatory assistance is required.

Treatment of these infants with digitalis preparations has not been effective, and surgery to close the ductus has often been necessary and usually has resulted in rapid improvement. Prostaglandin synthesis inhibitors have been found to be effective in either closing or constricting the ductus arteriosus in premature infants. Indomethacin has been used most frequently; in most infants, the drug has been administered by orogastric tube, either in suspension or in an alkaline solution [16, 17]. More recently a lyophilized preparation for intravenous use has become available for clinical trials. The drug is administered in doses of 0.2 mg/kg every 8–12 h for a maximum of three doses. Clinical evidence of closure was noted in about 70 % of infants, and constriction, but not complete closure, was observed in another 15 %. Infants who have symptoms that are severe respond as frequently as those with milder symptoms. In view of the marked increase in the risk of renal complications in premature infants after indomethacin therapy in higher doses, or with continued administration, the individual dose and number of doses recommended above should not be exceeded.

With indomethacin therapy, urinary excretion usually decreases, but if oliguria is marked, the drug should be discontinued because anuria may develop. Also, if marked abdominal distension or reduced gastric emptying is noted, or if evidence of gastrointestinal bleeding occurs, the drug should be stopped because progression of symptoms may lead to severe necrotizing enterocolitis. Because of the potential renal complications, it is considered inadvisable to initiate indomethacin therapy in infants who have serum creatinine concentrations above 1.8–2.0 mg/dl. Also, because prostaglandin synthesis inhibitors interfere with platelet function, indomethacin should not be given if there is any evidence of bleeding. Possible long-term effects of indomethacin therapy in premature infants have not yet been assessed, but there does not appear to be any late adverse effect.

Recently, evidence suggests that indomethacin treatment is much more likely to be effective if it is administered early in the postnatal course. When given in the first few days after birth, there is a greater evidence of ductus closure than if therapy is delayed for 2–3 weeks. This has led to the suggestion that indomethacin should be administered to any premature infant, as soon as clinical evidence of ductus patency is manifest. This approach has, in one study with a relatively small number of patients, resulted in a reduction in duration of ventilatory assistance, in hospital stay, and in complications. Further clinical trials of this type are, however, indicated.

References

1   Reuss, M.L.; Rudolph, A.M.: Distribution and recirculation of umbilical and systemic venous blood flow in fetal lambs during hypoxia. J. Dev. Physiol. *2:* 71 (1980).
2   Rudolph, A.M.: Congenital diseases of the heart (Year Book Medical Publishers, Chicago 1974).
3   Sharpe, G.L.; Larsson, K.S.; Thalme, B.: Studies on the closure of the ductus arteriosus. XII. In utero effect of indomethacin and sodium salicylate in rats and rabbits. Prostaglandins *9:* 585 (1975).
4   Heymann, M.A.; Rudolph, A.M.: Effects of acetylsalicylic acid on the ductus arteriosus and circulation in fetal lambs in utero. Circulation Res. *38:* 418 (1976).
5   Terragno, N.A.; Terragno, A.: Prostaglandin metabolism in the fetal and maternal vasculature. Fed. Proc. *38:* 75 (1979).

6   Clyman, R.I.; Mauray, F.; Roman, C.; Rudolph, A.M.: PGE_1 is a more potent vasodilator of the lamb ductus arteriosus than is either PGI_2 or 6-keto-F_1-alpha. Prostaglandins *16:* 259 (1978).

7   Challis, J.R.G.; Dilley, S.R.; Robinson, J.S.; Thorburn, G.D.: Prostaglandins in the circulation of the fetal lamb. Prostaglandins *11:* 1041 (1976).

8   Clyman, R.I.; Mauray, F.; Heymann, M.A.; Rudolph, A.M.: Developmental responses of oxygen and indomethacin. Prostaglandins *15:* 993 (1978).

9   Heymann, M.A.; Rudolph, A.M.: Ductus arteriosus dilatation by prostaglandin E_1 in infants with pulmonary atresia. Pediatrics *59:* 325 (1977).

10 Silove, E.D.; Coe, J.Y.; Page, A.J.F.; Mitchell, M.D.: Long-term oral prostaglandin E_2 maintains patency of the ductus arteriosus (Abstract). Circulation *60:* II-6 (1979).

11 Heymann, M.A.; Berman, W., Jr.; Rudolph, A.M.; Whitman, V.: Dilatation of the ductus arteriosus by prostaglandin E_1 in aortic arch abnormalities. Circulation *59:* 169 (1979).

12 Rudolph, A.M.; Heymann, M.A.; Spitznas, U.: Hemodynamic considerations in the development of narrowing of the aorta. Am.J.Cardiol.*30:* 514 (1972).

13 Lewis, A.B.; Freed, M.D.; Heymann, M.A.; Roehl, S.L.; Chen Kensey, R.: Side effects of therapy with prostaglandin E_1 in infants with critical congenital heart disease. Circulation *64:* 393 (1981).

14 Gittenberger-de-Groot, A.C.; Moulaert, A.J.; Harinck, E.; Becker, A.E.: Histopathology of the ductus arteriosus after prostaglandin E_1 administration in ductus-dependent cardiac anomalies. Br.Heart J.*40:* 215 (1978).

15 Haworth, S.G.; Sauer, U.; Buhlmeyer, K.: Effects of prostaglandin E_1 on pulmonary circulation in pulmonary atresia. A quantitative morphometric study. Br.Heart J. *43:* 306 (1980).

16 Friedman, W.F.; Hirschklau, M.J.; Printz, M.P.; Pitlick, P.T.; Kirkpatrick, S.E.: Pharmacological closure of the patent ductus arteriosus in premature infants. New Engl.J.Med.*295:* 526 (1976).

17 Heymann, M.A.; Rudolph, A.M.; Silverman, N.H.: Closure of the ductus arteriosus in premature infants by inhibition of prostaglandin synthesis. New Engl.J.Med.*295:* 530 (1976).

Abraham M.Rudolph, MD, Department of Pediatrics, Obstetrics, Gynecology, and Reproductive Sciences, and Physiology, and Cardiovascular Research Institute, University of California, San Francisco, CA 94143 (USA)

Mod. Probl. Paediat., vol. 22, pp. 15–25 (Karger, Basel 1983)

Cardiomyopathies in Infancy

E. Rossi

Department of Pediatrics, University of Berne, Berne, Switzerland

There are only a few studies on cardiomyopathies (CM) in infancy. In 1954 we published a monography on cardiomegaly in infants and made a first attempt at differential diagnosis [26]. Further contributions to this type of disorders in pediatric age was given by *Gilliland and McNamara* [7], *Fiddler* et al. [6] and *Pernot* [20].

The classification of CM (fig. 1) as proposed in 1978 by *Goodwin* [8] – although incomplete and to some extent arbitrary – deserves the merit to have, at least as regards the didactic usefulness, brought some clarification into this complex topic. The author differentiates between *congestive (dilatative, hypokinetic) CM* (CCM) and *hypertrophic-obstructive CM* (HOCM), as well as between *HOCM with typical subaortic stenosis* and the *atypical form with medioventricular or apical obstruction*. There is further a *hypertrophic non-obstructive variant* (NOCM). In addition, we have to include *obliterative (constructive) forms* such as endocardial fibroelastosis, and CM representing *secondary manifestations* of other diseases.

The cardiopathies in infancy are characterized by: high familial incidence; frequent cardiomegaly; absence of murmurs or only slight murmur; absence of cyanosis; normal or low blood pressure; dyspnea; frequent arrhythmia; intracardial thrombosis; frequent sudden death.

The introduction of new diagnostic methods, especially the heart catheterization, heart angiocardiography, echocardiography, and finally biopsy have allowed one to elaborate a classification which is far from being sufficiently satisfactory but, especially from a didactical point of view, it may be a starting point for discussion (table I).

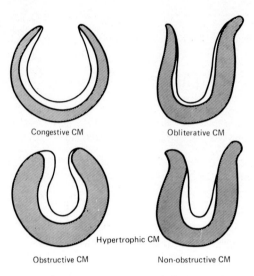

Congestive CM   Obliterative CM

Obstructive CM   Non-obstructive CM

Hypertrophic CM

Fig. 1. Classification of CM [modified after rep. 8].

Table I. Classification of Cardiomyopathies

I   Congestive (hypokinetic or dilatative) forms (CCM)
    (a)   Infectious
    (b)   Toxic
    (c)   Dysmetabolic

II Hypertrophic forms (HCM)
    (a)   Obstructive-functional hypertrophic form of subaortic stenosis (HOCM)
    (b)   Atypical form with medioventricular or apical obstruction
    (c)   Non-obstructive form (HNOCM)

III Obliterative, constrictive forms
    Fibroelastosis endocardica

IV Cardiomyopathies due to other diseases

Congestive or Hypokinetic Forms of Cardiomyopathy

Congestive or hypokinetic forms – also called, as was lately proposed, dilatative – may have an infectious, toxic or dysmetabolic origin. They are characterized by dilatation of the left ventricle, increase of the residual telesystolic and telediastolic volume and, consequently, a diminished systolic ejection and cardiac output. The cardiac hypertrophy is not very pronounced and the difference between contraction of the systole and diastole is only small. The *etiology* is most often unknown; it may be a viral infection or an autoimmune disease. *Clinically*, one may register dyspnea, palpitation after exercise, gallop rhythm, arrhythmia, auricular fibrillation, syncope, thromboembolism, and sometimes a systolic murmur due to mitral valve insufficiency [29]. The *ECG* may reveal an absence of signs of hypertrophy, left deviation of the axis QRS, and possibly a left branch block and total arrhythmia.

The *diagnosis* can only be made with certainty with the help of invasive methods. Decisive for diagnosis are dilatation of the ventricles and reduction of the contractions. The clinical importance of myocardial biopsy is a controversial issue. *Kunkel* [13], in over 200 biopsies of the left ventricle, found in congestive forms mostly muscular hypertrophy combined with interstitial proliferation. *Richardson and Atkinson* [23] measured several enzyme activities in biopsy samples and found no differences between patients with CM and those with valvular heart diseases showing left ventricular dysfunction. Higher levels of enzyme activity may more often be observed in cases with myocardial damage, such as the one caused by alcohol, but may also reflect the degree of hypertrophy. According to *Bolte* [2] immunological findings may be helpful in understanding various pathogenetic mechanisms of dilatative CM.

Prognosis is severe, especially if an important hemodynamic left ventricular insufficiency was observed at the time of the diagnosis. *Kuhn* et al. [12], based on a 8-year observation of 258 patients, reported a lethality rate of 80%. A correlation with findings made at biopsy revealed that the collective of patients with moderate morphological changes has a 6-year survival rate of 47% (n = 62). Death may be due to progressive heart failure, total arrhythmias and/or thromboembolism. So far, statistical evaluations were based principally on adults, but recent observations show an increasing number of such cases also in children and adolescents.

The *treatment*, therefore, includes antifailure, antiarrhythmic and anti-coagulant therapy [30]. *Digitalis* is indicated especially when auricular fibrillation with high ventricular rate is present. *Diuretica* are the standard drugs in cases of heart failure but they do not improve the ejection fraction or the cardiac output. *Spirolactone* is particularly helpful. *Vasodilatating agents*, such as an angiotensin-converting enzyme (Captopril = Lopirin®), are more and more being employed with good results. Captopril was also successfully used by *Riegger* et al. [25]. Positive results reportedly obtained with *Phentolamin Retard* and with *Dihydralazin* were not confirmed by other authors

[5, 15, 22]. A new β_1-antagonist, *Prenalterol*, is still in the experimental phase, but seems to be useful [11, 14].

Primary Hypertrophic Cardiomyopathies

In the group of primary hypertrophic CM one distinguishes *obstructive* and *non-obstructive* variants. Recent observations have indicated that, besides the hypertrophic obstructive forms with typical subaortal stenosis, atypical conditions with medioventricular and apical obstruction also exist. Classical and well-documented is the finding of a myocardial hypertrophy of unknown origin, especially an asymmetrical hypertrophy of the interventricular septum and, as a consequence, an insufficient 'compliance' of the left ventricle with or without an obstacle to ejection. Rarely, as pointed out by Italian authors [3, 4], it may also be localized in the right ventricle.

Obstructive Functional Hypertrophic Form of Subaortic Stenosis

The obstructive form is mainly seen in young adults, but there are many cases of pediatric age as well, even in infancy [17]. In contrast to earlier postulates, most authors now believe that the asymmetric hypertrophy of the interventricular septum has a genetic origin and that is followed by a functional obstruction of the ventricular ejection [21]. *Pernot* [20] reported on 143 patients, aged between 2 days and 20 years, with septal hypertrophic myopathies, among which 59 were obstructive. The author underlines a prevalence of the male sex, that their occurrence is highly familial and in an association with malformations. In infants the evolution is especially malignant. Often the asymmetrical hypertrophy of the ventricular septum involves the aortic and even the mitral valve, so that an insufficiency of the latter may be part of the condition.

From a *physiological* point of view, one usually notices a reduction of the left ventricle compliance with diminished diastolic distension, and an augmentation of the telesystolic pressure, often combined with a diminution of the telediastolic volume and of the ejection fraction. As a consequence, one can observe an increased pressure in the left atrium, a dilatation of the left atrium and – at times – atrial fibrillations.

Histological findings have been described in many studies based on biopsies; however, so far this was done only in adults. Obstructive CM are very often familial. They appear to be transmitted following an autosomal dominant trait. The hypothesis of an abnormal persistance of the primordial cardiac bulb, which physiologically is destined to involute on the left side, has been forwarded.

Clinically, symptoms may be completely lacking, especially in infants and small children. Often one registers dyspnea, precordial pain, paroxysmal tachycardia, vertigo, syncope and total arrhythmia. In cases with mitral valve insufficiency a typical murmur is heard. With a few exceptions of typical HOCM the definitive diagnosis can only be made using invasive methods. The intraventricular systolic pressure gradient is particularly important.

The echocardiogram may be essential for diagnosis. One usually observes a diminished telediastolic and telesystolic diameter of the left ventricle, an asymmetrical thickening of the interventricular septum, a stenosis of the ejection tract and – sometimes – mitral valve insufficiency. In some cases the echocardiographic changes are non-specific; however, together with the systolicum and the double-peak carotic pulse, they are important for diagnosis.

Radiologically, cardiomegaly is very frequent, especially in infants. Angiocardiography confirms the characteristic manifestations observed in the echocardiogram, i.e. the convex aspect of the interventricular septum protruding into the right ventricle. In the majority of cases, as pointed out by *Pernot* [20], it is possible to detect a systolic intraventricular gradient. Heart catheterization and perhaps sonography [24] are important in cases in which surgical intervention is considered.

The Atypical Forms with Medioventricular or Apical Obstruction Are Diagnosed by Invasive Methods.

Hypertrophic Non-Obstructive Forms

Primary hypertrophic 'non-obstructive' CM, in contrast to earlier reports, are as frequent as the obstructive forms, especially in the pediatric age groups. The telediastolic and the telesystolic diameter is diminished or normal; however, there is a typical absence of symptoms connected with an obstacle to ventricular ejection. In addition, these CM exhibit a slow and progressive evolution and may be followed by sudden death although, according to *Pernot* [20], they are not as frequent as in the obstructive forms (7 versus 14 %). Abnormally pointed negative T waves in the ECG seem to be important for diagnosis. The familial incidence, based on 49 cases observed by *Kuhn* et al. [12], was 15 %.

The *therapy* of obstructive and non-obstructive forms of primary hypertrophic CM may be medical and/or surgical. Treatment with *β-blocking agents*, such as propranolol, has improved the prognosis in the acute and subacute phase, less in the so long term. The recently introduced calcium antagonist *Verapamil* provides for a more successful therapy. *Kaltenbach* et al. [9], administering a dose of 480 mg orally, observed in 50 patients improvement lasting up to 7 years. The surgical treatment consists in myomectomy in the obstructive form and, if an insufficiency of the mitral valve is present, in valve substitution. According to *Pilotti* et al. [21] the therapeutical line to follow may be summarized as follows:

First stage   gradient between ventricle and aorta under 50 mm Hg in asymptomatic patients: no treatment
Second stage   gradient between 40 and 90 mm Hg in patients with symptoms: medical treatment with propranolol
Third stage   gradient of 90 mm Hg in individuals with severe symptoms: myomectomy and perhaps valve substitution

Senning and Rothlin [27] have noticed improvement in 41 out of 44 adult patients. A relapse was observed in 10 cases inasmuch as the disease progressed despite myotomy. *Binet* [1] presented similar, very good results obtained in 100 adults and he now has some experiences with children.

Obliterative, Constrictive Form

Of this group, I shall give especial consideration to endocardial fibroelastosis (table II). One may distinguish a primary form, especially the important true infantile variant, and secondary forms which are combined with heart malformations or dysmetabolic diseases, mainly of the neuromuscular type. From a hemodynamic point of view, both these forms are characterized by a diminished capacity of the heart to expand, i.e. an insufficient telediastol and incomplete inotropism. The heart shows a diffuse fibrous endocardial thickening with progressive narrowing of the ventricular cavity. In 90 % of cases, the change is localized in the left ventricle. The lesion often involves the mitral and the aortic valves. In such cases, implantation of valves may be followed by improvement of the clinical manifestations. The recent introduction of myocardial biopsies may help to establish the diagnosis which, until now, was only suspected.

Table II. Classification of endocardial fibroelastosis

Primary forms	Idiopathic infantile fibroelastosis
	Parietal endocarditis (Löffler)
	Cardiovascular collagenosis (Becker)
	Endomyocardial fibrosis (Davies)
Secondary forms	Combined with other malformations of the heart or with dysmetabolic disorders, especially neuromuscular diseases

Table III. Secondary cardiomyopathies

1 Forms with well-known etiology
  Infectious diseases (e.g. myocarditis)
  Toxic effects
  Nutritional deficiencies (e.g. selenium)
  Anemia
  Hormonal disturbances
  Conditions after prolonged assisted respiration in preterm babies

2 Forms with genetic origin
  (a) Mutants of only one gene
      Dysmetabolic disorders (e.g. glycogen storage diseases
      Pleismorphism of a mutant gene (e.g. lentiginosis, tuberous sclerosis
      Neuromuscular diseases
      Pancreatic diseases (e.g. cystic fibrosis)
  (b) Chromosomal anomalies
  (c) Abnormal mitochondria [18]
  (d) Conditions with a multifactorial etiology
      Cardiac malformations
      Neurocutaneous Kawasaki syndrome
      Cardiac tumors

Cardiomyopathies Due to Other Diseases: Secondary Cardiomyopathies

Among the group of secondary CM there are forms with well-known etiology and several variants of genetic origin [28]. We hope that the introduction of endomyocardial biopsy will allow us to expand our knowledge in this broad field. The secondary CM (table III) may lead to congestive or hypertrophic changes of the heart. It is impossible to discuss here all the different types known. Myopathies with well-known etiology comprise, for

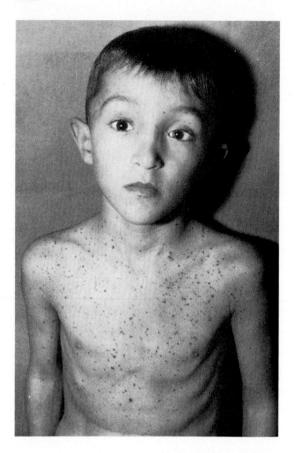

Fig. 2. R.F., male, born 5.11.1956. Lentiginosis and HOCM.

example, toxic forms such as those observed after treatment with adriamicin and daunomycin.

Among the cases due to 'alimentary deficiency', a cardiopathy with lethal evolution, which was recently observed mainly in Chinese people following an insufficient uptake of selenium, deserves special mention. This disease [10] seems to be caused by a deficit of glutamic peroxidase activity. The treatment with selenomethionine has allowed improvement in 82% of the cases.

Among the genetic forms, generalized glycogenoses are in the forefront. The increased glycogen content of muscles, the heart and – often – the central nervous system, results in a severe hypotonia, heart insufficiency and macroglossia. Clinically, these conditions may be subject to diagnostic difficulties, e.g. in separating them from Down's syndrome and hypothyroidism.

Particular interest was raised by the association of an obstructive hypertrophic CM with a neuroectodermic disease [16]. This syndrome is called *cardiopathic lentiginosis*. In children it is associated with deafness, hypogenitalism and psychosomatic infantilism. The transmission is mainly autosomal dominant. An Italian boy was admitted to our Children's Hospital in Berne in 1963 at the age of 6 years. He presented the typical picture of lentiginosis and HOCM confirmed by catheterization and surgical treatment (fig. 2).

Speaking of genetic forms, it is worthwhile remembering the CM observed in recent years in *cystic fibrosis*. These conditions may have a fatal outcome even in newborn and young infants and without any clinical manifestations of the disease. The pathogenesis may involve insufficient intestinal absorption of unknown substances important for myocardial metabolism. Another theory postulates the liberation of proteolytic enzymes, perhaps connected with the destruction of the exocrine pancreas, with consecutive activation of phlogistic substances, especially kinins [19].

The present short review, of necessity, was incomplete. However, I aimed at drawing the attention of cardiologists, particularly pediatric cardiologists, on this very complex chapter of CM in which so many problems still await further elucidation.

References

1   Binet, P.: Personal communication.
2   Bolte, H.-D.: Immunologische Untersuchungen bei dilativer Kardiomyopathie. Z. Kardiol. *70:* 606 (1981).
3   Botti, G.; Tagliavini, S.; Bonatti, V.; Aurier, E.: Isolated hypertrophic obstructive cardiomyopathy of the right ventricle. G. ital.Cardiol.*9:* 170–181 (1979).
4   Casanova, M.; Gamallo, C.; Quero-Jiménez, M.; García-Aguado, A.; Burgueros, M.; García, S.; Suarez, A.: Familial hypertrophic cardiomyopathy with unusual involvement of the right ventricle. Eur.J.Cardiol. *9:* 145–159 (1979).
5   Emb, W.; Mlczoch, J.: Phenolamin Retard bei Patienten mit kongestiver Kardiomyopathie. Z. Kardiol. *70:* 613 (1981).
6   Fiddler, G.I.; Tajik, A.J.; Weidmann, W.A.; McGoon, D.C.; Ritter, D.G.; Giuliani, E.R.: Idiopathic hypertrophic subaortic stenosis in the young. Am.J.Cardiol. *42:* 793–799 (1978).
7   Gilliland, J.C.; McNamara, D.G.: Idiopathic hypertrophic subaortic stenosis in children. Am.J.Cardiol.*21:* 99 (1968).

8   Goodwin, J.F.: Congestive and hypertrophic cardiomyopathies. A decade of study. Lancet *i:* 731–739 (1970).

9   Kaltenbach, M.; Hopf, R.; Kober, G.: Konservative medikamentöse Behandlung der hypertrophen Kardiomyopathien (HCM). Z. Kardiol. *70:* 624 (1981).

10   Keshan Disease Research Group of the Chinese Academy of Medical Sciences, Beijing: Epidemiologic studies on the etiologic relationship of selenium and Keshan disease. Chinese med. J. *92:* 477–482 (1979).

11   Kment, A.; Motz, W.; Ringsgwandl, G.; Kühnl, B.E.; Strauer, B.E.: Langzeitwirkung von Prenalterol bei dilatativer Cardiomyopathie. Z. Kardiol. *70:* 614 (1981).

12   Kuhn, H.; Thelen, U.; Köhler, E.; Lösse, B.: Die hypertrophische nicht obstruktive Kardiomypathie (HNCM) – klinische, hämodynamische, elektro-, echo- und angiokardiographische Untersuchungen. Z. Kardiol. *69:* 457–469 (1980).

13   Kunkel, K.: Morphologische Untersuchungen von Myokardbiopsien bei kongestiver Kardiomyopathie und ihre klinische Bedeutung. Z. Kardiol. *70:* 605 (1981).

14   Lambertz, H.; Erbel, R.; Meyer, J.; Schweizer, P.; Effert, E.: Langzeitergebnisse in der Behandlung von schweren kongestiven Kardiomyopathien (COCM) mit dem neuen β_1-Agonisten Prenalterol (P). Z. Kardiol. *70:* 614 (1981).

15   Manthey, J.; Dietz, R.; Ke, N.Y.; Leinberger, H.; Mäurer, W.; Schömig, A.; Schwarz, F.; Kübler, W.: Reflektorische Zunahme der sympatho-neuronalen Aktivität nach Hydralazin bei Patienten mit congestiver Cardiomyopathie (CoCMP). Z. Kardiol. *70:* 613 (1981).

16   Moynahan, E.J.; Polani, P.: Progressive profuse lentiginosis, progressive cardiomyopathy, short stature with delayed puberty, mental retardation or psychic infantilism, and other developmental anomalies: a new familial syndrome; in Jadassohn, Schirren, 13th Congr. Int. Dermatologiae, vol. 2, pp. 1543–1544 (Springer, Berlin 1968).

17   Neufeld, H.N.; Ongley, P.A.; Edwards, J.E.: Combined congenital subaortic stenosis and infundibular pulmonary stenosis. Br. Heart J. *22:* 686–690 (1960).

18   Neustein, H.B.; Lurie, P.R.; Dahms, B.; Takahashi, M.: An X-linked recessive cardiomyopathy with abnormal mitochondria. Pediatrics, Springfield *64:* 24–29 (1979).

19   Nezelof, C.; LeSec, G.: Multifocal myocardial necrosis and fibrosis in pancreatic diseases of children. Pediatrics, Springfield *63:* 361–368 (1979).

20   Pernot, C.: Myocardiopathie obstructive du nourrisson, de l'enfant et de l'adolescent. A propos de 59 observations. Ann. Cardiol. Angélol. *29:* 159–169 (1980).

21   Pilotti, G.; Burzio, P.; Favetta, S.; Ricci, C.; Pennacino, G.: La cardiomiopatia ostruttiva con stenosi subaortica ipertrofica idiopatica in età pediatrica. Min. Med. *70:* 3299–3307 (1979).

22   Reifart, N.; Bunge, T.; Kaltenbach, M.; Bussmann, W.D.: Beschränkter Therapieerfolg bei Langzeitbehandlung der schweren kongestiven Kardiomyopathie mit Dihydralazin. Z. Kardiol. *70:* 613 (1981).

23   Richardson, P.J.; Atkinson, L.: Enzyme analysis of endomyocardial biopsies in congestive (dilated) cardiomyopathy. Z. Kardiol. *70:* 605 (1981).

24   Richter-Von Arnauld, H.P.; Sonntag, F.; Feigel, H.: Nichtinvasive hämodynamische Beurteilung der idiopathischen hypertrophischen Subaortenstenose mit der direktionalen Doppler-Sonographie. Z. Kardiol. *70:* 626 (1981).

25   Riegger, A.J.G.; Steilner, H.; Liebau, G.: Beziehungen zwischen Hämodynamik und Pressorhormonsystemen unter Captopril bei congestiver Cardiomyopathie. Z. Kardiol. *70:* 613 (1981).
26   Rossi, E.: Herzkrankheiten im Säuglingsalter (Thieme, Stuttgart 1954).
27   Senning, Å.; Rothlin, M.: Chirurgie bei hypertropher obstruktiver Kardiomyopathie. Z. Kardiol. *70:* 625 (1981).
28   Takao, A.; Nishikawa, T.; Takarada, M.: Secondary cardiomyopathies in childhood. Jap. Circ. J. *43:* 1009–1016 (1979).
29   Vajola, S.F.; Lax, A.M.; Castellari, M.; Ceci, V.; Masini, V.: Osservazioni epidemiologiche e cliniche su 300 casi di miocardiopatie primitive. G. ital. Cardiol. *9:* 434–437 (1979).
30   Waagstein, F.: Treatment of congestive cardiomyopathy. Z. Kardiol. *70:* 606 (1981).

Prof. Dr. E. Rossi, Universitäts-Kinderklinik, Inselspital, CH-3010 Bern (Schweiz)

Mod. Probl. Paediat., vol. 22, pp. 26–37 (Karger, Basel 1983)

Pediatric Nuclear Cardiology: Applications and Utility

M. S. Schaffer, M. E. de Souza, D. L. Gilday, R. D. Rowe

Divisions of Cardiology (Department of Paediatrics) and Nuclear Medicine (Department of Radiology), The Hospital for Sick Children, University of Toronto, Faculty of Medicine, Toronto, Ontario, Canada

Applications

Although nuclear medicine has evolved from the humble scintillation probe to sophisticated gamma camera computer processing of scintigraphic data over 50 years, its routine use in pediatric cardiology has occurred in only the past 5 years. It is the newer developments in computer technology that have made application to this age group feasible.

This review looks at specific applications, current developments and utility of radionuclide techniques in pediatric cardiology. In addition it concentrates on assessment of problems with surgical implications.

These applications include evaluations of intracardiac shunting, the anatomy of venous connections, the distribution of pulmonary blood flow through obstructions or interruptions, ventricular function and myocardial infarction.

Radionuclide angiocardiography, gated equilibrium blood pool analysis and myocardial scintigraphy are the three main techniques used in pediatric nuclear cardiology. Our experience with more than 1,400 studies using these methods (table I) in nuclear medicine and cardiology at the Hospital for Sick Children, Toronto, since 1973 forms the basis of this report. The patients ranged in age from newborn to 26 years (fig. 1).

Radionuclide Angiocardiography

The radioactive bolus injected intravenously is followed through the heart, much in the manner of the venous contrast cineangiocardiogram. The patient is positioned supine under a gamma camera with a high-sensitivity collimator so that the heart and right lung are in the field of view. ^{99m} Tc in

Table I. Radionulide studies performed at The Hospital For Sick Children from 1973 to 1981

Study	Number
Angiocardiograms	729
Gated equilibrium blood pool imaging	323
Myocardial perfusion scintigrams	389
Total	1,441

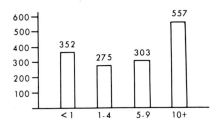

Fig. 1. Nuclear cardiovascular procedures, grouped by patient age, at The Hospital for Sick Children, Toronto, 1973–1981.

the form of sodium pertechnate is administered by rapid intravenous bolus at a dose of 215 μCi/kg ($<$15 kg body wt) or 285 μCi/kg ($\pm$15 kg body wt) and images are acquired at four frames per second for 40 s. This allows the tracer to be followed through the cardiac chambers, while delivering only a modest radiation dose to the patient [1].

Radionuclide angiograms can delineate abnormal intracardiac connections [2]. Recently, computer assisted analysis has enhanced image resolution and improved diagnostic capabilities in the cyanotic infant [3].

Delineation of venous connections in specific instances can be most helpful. Identification of and assessment of the patency of single or bilateral superior venae cavae are necessary in the pre- and postoperative assessment of Glenn or Fontan-type procedures (fig. 2). Vena caval obstruction after repair of sinus venosus atrial septal defect or Mustard intra-atrial baffle procedures can be demonstrated in this fashion [4]. Also, this technique may be used to screen the state of the larger lung vessels obstructed on the arterial or venous side by demonstrating differences in distribution of flow (fig. 3).

At present, the most common use of radionuclide angiograms is to generate time-activity curves from the passage of the radioactive bolus

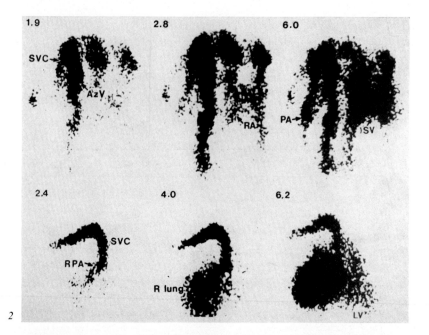

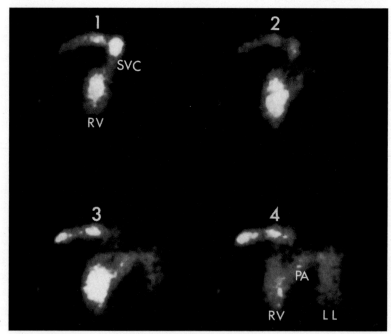

through the circulation. Areas of interest over the superior vena cava and right lung are defined, permitting creation of time-activity curves analogous to indicator-dilution curves (figs. 4, 5). First the adequacy of the bolus must be established (a smooth, continuous flow lasting less than 3 s in the superior vena cava) and then the magnitude of an intracardiac shunt may be quantified.

After quantifying left-to-right shunting, *Askenazi* et al. [5] found a correlation coefficient of 0.94 between radionuclide angiograms and catheterization oximetry. In our experience, the correlation is 0.82 [unpublished data] while *McIlveen* et al. [6] reported a correlation of 0.71 when the pulmonary to systemic flow ratio was between 1.0 and 3.0.

One of the most important applications of nuclear cardiology is in evaluating shunts at the atrial level, especially those whose size makes the need for surgical intervention borderline. Postoperatively, it is quite helpful in patients with clinical signs of a residual shunt. In complex anomalies, where a murmur may be related to a shunt or valvar regurgitation, it is somewhat less helpful.

The most frequent source of error in assessing shunts is a bolus that moves slowly and erratically through the superior vena cava, as depicted by the time activity curve. Use of short-lived radiopharmaceuticals such as oxygen-labeled carbon dioxide that avoid the need for the cumbersome jugular injection and do not depend on patient cooperation would be preferable [7].

The rôle of nuclear techniques in preterm infants who have cardiac defects with left-to-right shunting is much less clear. In these children, about whom little clinical doubt exists concerning the necessity of surgery, it is important to define the number and position of such defects. This information is best obtained through echocardiography and contrast cineangiocardiography [8, 9].

Fig. 2. Two venous angiograms. The lower three frames show passage of the technetium bolus from the superior vena cava (SVC) to the right pulmonary artery (RPA) and right lung in a patient with a patent Glenn anastomosis. The upper three frames show a patient in whom the Glenn anastomosis is partially obstructed. There is collateral flow through the azygous vein (AzV) into the right atrium (RA) and the single ventricle (SV). (Courtesy of Dr. *H. Wesselhoeft*).

Fig. 3. Pulmonary counts confined to the left lung in a patient with right pulmonary venous obstruction. LL = Left lung; PA = pulmonary artery; RV = right ventricle; SVC = superior vena cava.

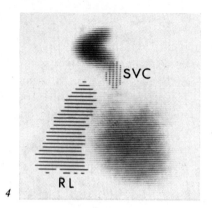

4

SVC

R L

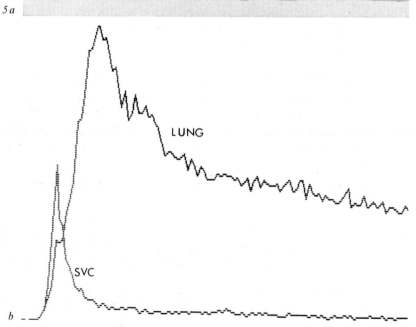

LUNG

5 a

LUNG

SVC

b

Equilibrium Blood Pool Imaging

In gated equilibrium blood pool imaging, multiple images are obtained during the cardiac cycle and played back in a continuous loop cineventriculogram. Red blood cells are labeled in vivo by injecting stannous pyrophosphate (0.4 mg/kg body wt) followed 20 min later by injection of ^{99m}Tc pertechnate in the same dose as for an angiogram. After equilibration of the technetium in the blood pool, a gamma camera with a high-resolution slant hole collimator is positioned for the 45° left anterior oblique view. A 10–20° caudal angulation is used to ensure the best delineation and separation of the cardiac chambers. Each cardiac cycle is divided into frames. The corresponding frames for all the cycles are then summed to produce an equilibrium ventriculogram of the sequential frames (fig. 6).

Regions of interest may be defined as in angiography. Time-activity curves can then be constructed and ejection fraction and relative ventricular volumes calculated as follows:

$$EF = \frac{EDC - ESC,}{EDC}$$

where EF = ejection fraction, EDC = end-diastolic counts and ESC = end-systolic counts. From the ventricular volume curves, one can also examine contractility (peak rate of ejection) and diastolic compliance (peak rate of ventricular filling) [10]. Wall motion can be assessed both qualitatively and by comparing computed ejection fractions for various ventricular segments [11].

Perhaps the most important pediatric use to date of gated equilibrium studies has been in assessing ventricular function. This type of study is important in cardiomyopathies but also offers a way to follow ventricular function in many of the major congenital anomalies before and after surgery. Such studies have been useful in evaluating pre- and postoperative valvar regurgitation [12].

Serial studies of ventricular function at rest and with exercise are now routinely available. In our unit, *Benson* et al. [13] and *Harder* et al. [14] have

---

Fig. 4. Computer-constructed regions of interest over the superior vena cava (SVC) and right lung (RL). The time acting curve constructed from the region over the superior vena cava is used to assess the adequacy of the bolus injection. The curve from the region over the right lung is used to evaluate the pulmonary circulation (see text).

Fig. 5. Time-activity curves in patients with (*a*) no shunting, (*b*) large left-to-right shunting.

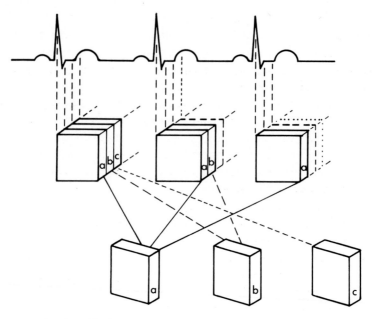

Fig.6. Gated equilibrium cineventriculogram (see text).

used changes in ejection fraction from rest to exercise to assess ventricular function in patients with complete transposition of the arteries [13] and tricuspid atresia [14]. The effects of exercise on ventricular function are now being evaluated at our institution in children who have hyperlipedemia. Also, radionuclides have been used in assessing the cardiac function of patients with pulmonary disease [15]. We are currently using these techniques to evaluate the effects of pharmacologic intervention in children with cystic fibrosis.

Myocardial Perfusion Scintigraphy

Myocardial scintigraphic imaging became a popular method for assessing myocardial ischemia and infarction in 1973. Since 1975, ^{201}Tl, a potassium analogue, which is cyclotron produced, has been employed as a radionuclide marker [16]. Its distribution depends on blood flow and cellular uptake and release. Therefore, scintigraphic images correspond to myocardial perfusion and viability.

Ischemia and infarction are differentiated on the basis of redistribution [17]. Immediately after injection, both lesions display decreased uptake;

however, 4–6 h later, ischemic areas are filled in while infarcted regions remain 'cold'.

Before imaging, patients are fasted 4 hours to decrease gastric uptake. ^{201}Tl is injected intravenously and imaging is performed immediately in the left anterior oblique, left lateral and anterior views. A high-resolution converging or parallel-hole collimator is used for image enhancement. Regions of interest are created over various segments of the myocardium and compared for accumulated radioactivity.

All of our experience with myocardial perfusion imaging has been using ^{201}Tl. In patients with suspected transient myocardial ischemia, the heart and lung are imaged in the anterior view to show the relationship between myocardial and pulmonary uptake. *Finley* et al. [18] showed that thallium uptake is decreased globally in neonates with transient myocardial ischemia and then improves over a 4- to 6-weeks recovery period.

Thallium perfusion studies can demonstrate myocardial infarction in patients with anomalous left coronary artery arising from the pulmonary artery [19, 20], or coronary arteritis. Also the severity of right ventricular hypertrophy and pulmonary hypertension may be estimated from the degree of right ventricular activity. These changes may be present earlier than other clinical parameters of cor pulmonale [21].

To date, myocardial perfusion studies in children have been somewhat disappointing. While infarctions may be significant, they are usually subendocardial and not well delineated with thallium scanning. This seems an area where other approaches now being developed, such as emission computed tomography, may prove helpful.

Current Developments

The newest developments include investigation of right ventricular function, assessment of regional wall motion, emission computed tomography and ultrashort half-life radiopharmaceuticals.

Analysis of right ventricular function is complicated by overlapping images from adjacent structures. In adults, good results have been obtained when the anterior view and a first-pass technique are used to isolate the various chambers for subsequent individual evaluation [15]. Also, the use of ^{81m}Kp, a radioactive gas eliminated in the lungs, has permitted equilibrium imaging of the right heart without left ventricular overlap [22]. In addition, we have used temporal Fourier analysis to distinguish between the atria and ventricles, based on differences of phase angles and amplitude [23].

Improved evaluation of regional wall motion is particularly important

for patients with coronary artery disease but it can also be applied for pre-
and postoperative assessments in those who have congenital heart malformations. The ventricle is divided into a number of segments and ejection
fractions may then be calculated for the different segments [11]. Alternatively,
the motion of the outlines of the ventricular cavity during contraction may
be analyzed. Irregular contraction patterns may also be investigated using
temporal Fourier analysis [24].

New, short-lived radiopharmaceuticals are particularly useful in pediatrics. They deliver a low radiation dose and can be repeated almost immediately because there is little background accumulation [25]. Oxygen-
labeled carbon dioxide ($0–15–CO_2$) seems especially promising since it can
be delivered by inhalation, avoiding the undesirable venipuncture [7].

Utility

It is important to determine the rôle of nuclear cardiology in pediatric
clinical assessment compared with the other resources available. For
example, echocardiography increasingly supplements clinical evaluation
while cardiac catheterization and angiography are still widely used for detailed diagnosis.

Nuclear techniques are becoming important tools for assessing complex
lesions, particularly in delineating patterns of venous connections and in
evaluating ventricular function at rest and with exercise. In contrast, it has
little rôle in evaluating obstructive lesions and cannot compare with other
approaches for assessing the severity of stenoses (table II).

While it is difficult to evaluate the additional benefit obtained from new
investigations in such a rapidly changing area as cardiac diagnosis, it is
necessary to compare the utility and cost of various procedures, beginning
with the chest roentgenograph as the simplest tool and including echocardiography, nuclear cardiology and cardiac catheterization with contrast
cineangiography. We still regard catheterization as the gold standard but it
has significant penalties in terms of complications, radiation dose and cost
(table II). The disadvantages of nuclear cardiology, which are radiation
dose and cost, are only modest at present.

It would be inappropriate to decide which is the best pediatric cardiovascular investigation. These tests are not used in isolation nor should they
be evaluated as such, but rather according to how they complement each
other. At present, echocardiography and catheterization are better suited to

Table II. Comparison of utility and cost in pediatric cardiovascular investigations

	Chest roentgenograph	Echocardio- graphy	Nuclear cardiology	Catheterization angiogram
Utility				
Shunt	fair	fair-good	good-excellent	excellent
Obstruction	poor	fair-good	poor	excellent
Complex disorder	fair	good	fair[1]	excellent
Ventricular function	poor	fair-good	excellent	excellent
Infarction	poor	fair	good-excellent	good
Cost				
Complications	0	0	0	+
Radiation dose, rad	0.024	0	0.5	1.0
Expense	low	medium	medium	high

[1] These techniques of estimating ventricular volumes and function have not as yet been validated.

defining anatomy and hemodynamics, while nuclear cardiology provides a safe, noninvasive method of evaluating and following intracardiac shunting and ventricular function at rest and with exercise. As the sophistication of nuclear cardiology increases, further analyses of utility will be needed to establish its role in pediatric cardiology.

References

1   Kereiakes, J.C.; Feller, P.A.; Ascoli, F.A.: Pediatric radiopharmaceutical dosimetry; in Cloutier, et al., Radiopharmaceutical Dosimetry Symp. Proc. Conf., Oak Ridge 1976. HEW Publ. (FDA) 76-8044, June 1976, pp. 77–91.

2   Wesselhoeft, H.; Hurly, P.J.; Wagner, H.N., Jr.; Rowe, R.D.: Nuclear angiocardiography in the diagnosis of congenital heart disease in infants. Circulation 45: 77–91 (1972).

3   Wesselhoeft, H.; Luig, H.; Emrich, D.; Galal, O.; Tacke, E.: Computer assisted nuclear angiocardiography in newborn infants. Technical improvement and results. Wld Congr. of Pediat. Cardiol., London 1980 (abstract 173).

4   Howman-Giles, R.B.; Gilday, D.L.; Mason, D.T.; Berman, D.S.: Nuclear cardiology in pediatrics: evaluation of intracardiac shunts and additional congenital disorders; in Berman, Mason, Clinical nuclear cardiology, pp. 285–317 (Grune & Stratton, New York, 1981).

5   Askenazi, J.; Ahnberg, D.S.; Korngold, E.; LaFarge, C.G.; Maltz, D.L.; Treves, S.:
     Quantitative radionuclide angiocardiography: detection and quantitation of left to
     right shunts. Am.J.Cardiol.*37:* 382–387 (1976).
6   McIlveen, B.M.; Hoschl, R.; Murray, I.P.; McCredie, R.M.; Chidiac, P.; Marriott,
     D.; Beveridge, J.: Radionuclide quantitation of left-to-right cardiac shunts in
     children. Aust. N.Z. J.Med.*8:* 500–508 (1978).
7   Tamer, D.M.; Watson, D.D.; Kenny, P.J.; Janowitz, W.R.; Gelband, H.; Gilson,
     A.J.: Noninvasive detection and quantification of left-to-right shunts in children using
     oxygen-15 labeled carbon dioxide. Circulation *56:* 626–631 (1977).
8   Bierman, F.Z.; Fellows, K.; Williams, R.G.: Prospective identification of ventri-
     cular septal defects in infancy using subxiphoid two-dimensional echocardiography.
     Circulation *62:* 807–817 (1980).
9   Fellows, K.E.; Westerman, G.R.; Keane, J.F.: Angiography of multiple ventricular
     septal defects in infancy (Abstract). Circulation *64:* suppl.IV, p.18 (1981).
10   Bacharach, S.L.; Green, M.V.; Borer, J.S.; Ostrow, H.G.; Bonow, R.O.; Farkas,
     S.P.; Johnston, G.S.: Beat-by-beat validation of ECG gating. J.nucl.Med.*21:*
     307–313 (1980).
11   Uren, R.; Maddox, D.E.; Parker, J.A.; Idoine, J.; Cohn, P.F.; Holman, B.L.:
     Validation of regional ejection fraction: quantitative radionuclide assessment of
     regional left ventricular function (Abstract). Circulation *56:* suppl.III, p.61 (1977).
12   Hurwitz, R.A.; Treves, S.; Freed, M.: Radionuclide assessment of aortic and mitral
     regurgitation (Abstract). Circulation *64:* suppl.IV p.277 (1981).
13   Benson, L.N.; Bonet, J.; McLaughlin, P.; Olley, P.M.; Feiglin, D.; Druck, M.;
     Trusler, G.A.; Rowe, R.D.; Morch, J.: Assessment of right ventricular function
     during supine bicycle exercise after Mustard's operation. Circulation (in press).
14   Harder, J.R.; Gilday, D.L.; deSouza, M.; Freedom, R.M.; Olley, P.M.; Rowe,
     R.D.: Radionuclide assessment of left ventricular function in patients with tricuspid
     atresia (Abstract). Am.J.Cardiol.*47:* 431 (1981).
15   Berger, H.J.; Matthay, R.A.; Loke, J.; Marshall, R.C.; Gottschalk, A.; Zaret, B.L.:
     Assessment of cardiac performance with quantitative radionuclide angiocardio-
     graphy: right ventricular ejection fraction with reference to findings in chronic
     obstructive pulmonary disease. Am.J.Cardiol.*41:* 897–905 (1978).
16   Strauss, H.W.; Harrison, K.; Langan, J.K.; Lebowitz, E.; Pitt, B.: Thallium-201
     for myocardial imaging: relation of thallium-201 to regional myocardial perfusion,
     Circulation *51:* 641–645 (1975).
17   Pohost, G.M.; Zir, L.M.; Moore, R.H.; McKusick, K.A.; Guiney, T.E.; Beller,
     G.A.: Differentiation of transiently ischemic from infarcted myocardium by serial
     imaging after a single dose of thallium-201. Circulation *55:* 294–302 (1977).
18   Finley, J.P.; Howman-Giles, R.B.; Gilday, D.L.; Bloom, K.R.; Rowe, R.D.:
     Transient myocardial ischemia of the newborn infant demonstrated by thallium
     myocardial imaging. J.Pediat.*94:* 263–270 (1979).
19   Finley, J.P.; Howman-Giles, R.; Gilday, D.L.; Olley, P.M.; Rowe, R.D.: Thallium-
     201 myocardial imaging in anomalous left coronary artery arising from the pulmo-
     nary artery: applications before and after medical and surgical treatment. Am.J.
     Cardiol.*42:* 675–680 (1978).
20   Gutgesell, H.P.; Pinsky, W.W.; DePuey, E.G.: Thallium-201 myocardial perfusion

imaging in infants and children: value in distinguishing anomalous left coronary artery from congestive cardiomyopathy. Circulation *61:* 596–599 (1980).

21 Cohen, H.A.; Baird, M.G.; Rouleau, J.R.; Fuhrmann, C.F.; Bailey, I.K.; Summer, W.R.; Strauss, H.W.; Pitt, B.: Thallium 201 myocardial imaging in patients with pulmonary hypertension. Circulation *54:* 790–795 (1976).

22 Polcyn, R.E.; Nickles, R.J.: Experimental approaches to myocardial function studies: $C^{15}O_2$ and ^{81m}Kr. Semin.nucl.Med. *7:* 101–105 (1977).

23 Douglas, K.H.; Links, J.M.; Alderson, P.O.; Wagner, H.N.: Temporal Fourier analysis in the selection of right ventricular regions of interest. Proc. 10th Ann. Symp. Society of Nuclear Medicine Computer Council, Miami Beach 1980.

24 Links, J.M.; Douglas, K.H.; Wagner, H.N., Jr.: Patterns of ventricular emptying by Fourier analysis of gated blood-pool studies. J.nucl.Med. *21:* 978–982 (1980).

25 Chervu, L.R.: Radiopharmaceuticals in cardiovascular nuclear medicine. Semin. nucl.Med. *9:* 241–256 (1979).

Richard D.Rowe, MD, Professor of Paediatrics, University of Toronto, Director Division of Cardiology, The Hospital for Sick Children, Toronto, Ont. (Canada)

Mod. Probl. Paediat., vol. 22, pp. 38–47 (Karger, Basel 1983)

The Dynamic Spatial Reconstructor[1]

Erik L. Ritman

Biodynamics Research Unit, Mayo Foundation, Mayo Clinic, Mayo Graduate School of Medicine, Rochester, Minn,. USA

The dynamic spatial reconstructor (DSR) is a multiple X-ray source scanner which images a volume in a fraction of a second and repeats this scan many times per second [1, 2]. It was designed and built with funds primarily from grants of the US government's National Institutes of Health. An artist's conception of the DSR is presented in figure 1. The subject lies on a horizontal table surrounded by a metal ring, to which are attached 14 X-ray tubes and an equal number of television cameras. The machine is 6 m long and 4.5 m in diameter and weighs about 15 tons. Figure 1b schematically indicates the data flow from the scanner to the operator interactive image analysis terminal. Installation was started in late 1979. The DSR scanner facility is illustrated in figures 2 and 3.

The purpose of the DSR is to make measurements more accurately than are currently possible using conventional non-invasive techniques. In addition, it is designed to make simultaneous measurements of structure and function. Whereas many conventional instruments can be used to make quite accurate, but isolated, measurements of structure or function, these isolated accurate measurements may be of little value when the simultaneous interrelationship of dynamic structure to function is of primary value.

The basic mechanism behind this machine is very similar to that of CAT scanners. A major reason for the use of the CAT scan principle is that this overcomes the superposition problem. It allows accurate measurements of internal structures, something that is generally not possible with certainty if projection imaging is used. However, commercial CAT scan

[1] This work was supported in part by research grants HL-04664 and RR-00007 from the National Institutes of Health.

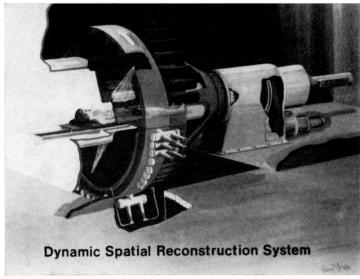

Dynamic Spatial Reconstruction System

a

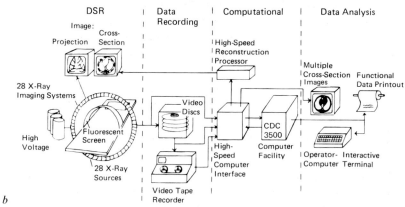

b

Fig. 1. a Artist's conception of DRS illustrating the multiple X-ray tubes and video cameras. *b* Flow chart of the data-processing sequence between the scanner (far left) and the operator-interactive data analysis system (far right) [from ref. 5 with permission].

systems are of limited use for scanning moving structures such as the heart, lungs, and circulation. First, a single scan requires several seconds to obtain, resulting in blurring because the heart beats once every second or so. Although gated scans can be used in some instances to minimize blurring, this technique does not permit accurate imaging of transient events. The DSR achieves rapid completion of a scan because each X-ray source is elec-

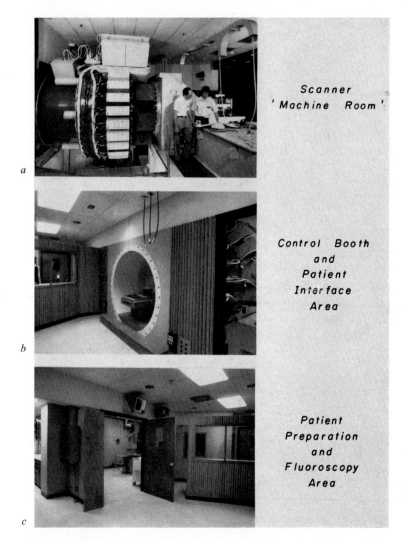

Scanner
'Machine Room'

Control Booth
and
Patient
Interface
Area

Patient
Preparation
and
Fluoroscopy
Area

Fig. 2. Three aspects of DSR scanner facility. *a* DSR scanner gantry. *b* Patient area
and control booth. Patient's head is visible in tunnel opening. *c* Conventional cardiac
catheterization laboratory with fluoroscopic system. This room is used primarily for
placement of catheters.

tronically pulsed for 350 μs – completing a 28-source scan in just under
11 ms. The high speed achieved minimizes image blurring due to heart beat,
breathing, or movement of blood or bowel. Secondly, commercial scanners

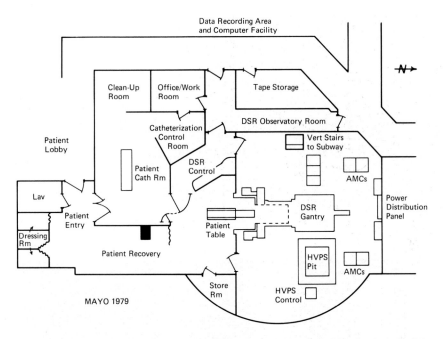

Fig. 3. Floor plan of DSR scanner facility. Patient lobby is conventiently accessible to climate-controlled underground tunnel connecting the outpatient areas and hospital.

generally produce images of only one slice per scan. The DSR also differs from commercial scanners in that it synchronously scans a volume rather than a single slice.

The DSR scans a cylindrical (22 cm diameter) volume within 0.01 s and generates up to 240 parallels, 1-mm thick, transverse sections. This capability is achieved as illustrated in figure 4. Being a television-based system, this procedure is repeated 60 times per second. This scan repetition rate enables the measurement of movement of blood (flow, perfusion) and air (ventilation). The basic image information generated by the DSR is illustrated in figure 5. In figure 5a is a conventional fluoroscopic image of the chest. Of the 240 parallel horizontal TV scan lines, 64 are brightened to show the location of the corresponding images of thin cross-sections generated in that one scan period. However, by themselves these images of transverse sections are often not very useful for quantitative analysis. This critically important point will be pursued further on in this manuscript.

Figure 6 shows a single CT image of a heart inside a dog. From pictures such as these, regional muscle wall thickness and time rates of change of

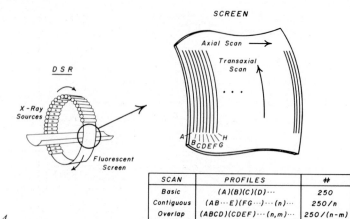

SCAN	PROFILES	#
Basic	$(A)(B)(C)(D)\cdots$	250
Contiguous	$(AB\cdots E)(FG\cdots)\cdots(n)\cdots$	$250/n$
Overlap	$(ABCD)(CDEF)\cdots(n,m)\cdots$	$250/(n-m)$

4

5 a   b

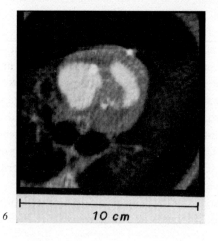

6

10 cm

wall thickness are measured. Such data, along with simultaneous chamber pressure, chamber area (index of chamber volume), are used to compute myocardial function and global ventricular function. Blood flow can also be estimated. Figure 7 illustrates how blood in a carotid artery flow was estimated. 2 or 4 ml of contrast agent were injected proximal to the imaged region. An electromagnetic flow meter at the distal end of the common carotid artery provided an independent estimate of flow. The entire neck was scanned but only two of the multiple 1-mm thick sections are illustrated. They are also shown in figure 7. Preliminary results indicate that area under the curve is inversely proportional to flow and directly proportional to the amount of contrast agent injected. These are necessary conditions for applying the Stewart-Hamilton formula to estimate flow. Comparison of the flow in the carotid artery as per flow meter with the flow as determined from the DSR data indicates that the DSR underestimated flow by 10%, a deviation to be expected from the indicator dilution technique. However, as increases in flow of up to several hundred percent following an intervention such as a vasodilator drug or exercise are to be expected if no vascular pathology is present, this accuracy is probably quite adequate for diagnostic purposes.

An important capability of the DSR is the accurate measurement of anatomic structure. As illustrated in figure 8, depending on the lesion or object of interest (a valve or a coronary artery or a piece of heart muscle), the slice of interest must be in the right place and the right orientation to allow accurate measurement. This orientation and location generally differs

---

Fig.4. The fluorescent screen is scanned by a television camera, one camera for each X-ray tube. Each television picture is made up of many horizontal scan lines. Each of these horizontal scan lines carries the information for one cross-section profile. The cameras generate, for each 0.01-second scan, up to 240 1-mm thick cross-sections. Retrospective addition of several adjacent horizontal video lines allows generation of images of slices of selected thickness, location, and spacing [from ref. 6 with permission].

Fig.5. a Roentgen image of a dog's chest generated by one of the multiple X-ray tubes and its corresponding TV camera. 64 of the up to 240 available horizontal locations for transverse images are indicated. *b* Images of transverse sections, each corresponding to a location indicated by the horizontal lines in the left panel. This stack of cross-sections can be generated within 0.01 second scan and repeated 60/second [from ref. 7 with permission].

Fig.6. Single transverse slice of heart in intact dog. Roentgen contrast agent (1 ml/kg) was injected intravenously. The two large bright areas are the left ventricular and right ventricular chambers. Myocardial mass and rate of wall thickness change can be evaluated from images of this and adjacent slices [from ref. 8 with permission].

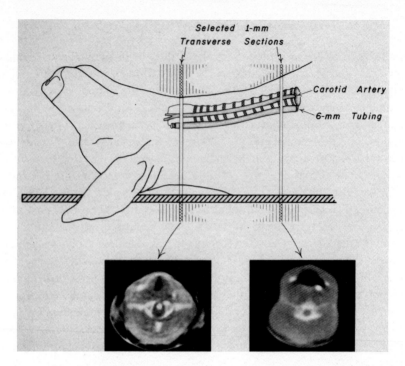

Fig. 7. Experimental verification that it is possible to estimate blood flow in carotid artery from passage of a bolus of roentgen contrast agent. Entire neck was scanned with DSR – two cross-section images are displayed. Brightness over carotid artery region was measured at 130-ms intervals over a 3-second period as a 2-ml bolus of contrast agent passed through artery. Tubing with known concentration contrast agent was surgically implanted parallel to carotid so as to provide a calibration [from ref. 9 with permission].

Fig. 8. Quantitative analysis of valve, orifice areas, myocardial wall thickness, and coronary artery diameters requires that images of oblique sections be computed from the stack of imaged parallel transverse sections. This process also requires that the location and orientation of the desired slice be visualized in relation to the 3-dimensional anatomy of the structure in a manner somewhat analogous to the central drawing in this figure.

Fig. 9. Roentgen contrast agent injected into the inferior vena cava passes through the right atrium and ventricle during a scan. Computer recognition of the blood/endo-cardial interface permits computation of the 3-dimensional shape of these chambers and associated large vessels. The lower panels represent four views of the same data at one instance in time during a cardiac cycle. These data permit estimation of chamber volume without the need to resort to simplifying assumptions as to chamber shape [from ref. 9 with permission].

Fig. 10. 3-dimensional surface display of myocardium of heart scanned in DSR. The right panel illustrates the capacity for 'non-invasive surgery'. From these images the complex anatomy can be evaluated and total muscle mass, regional wall thickness, and chamber volumes can be computed [from ref. 10 with permission].

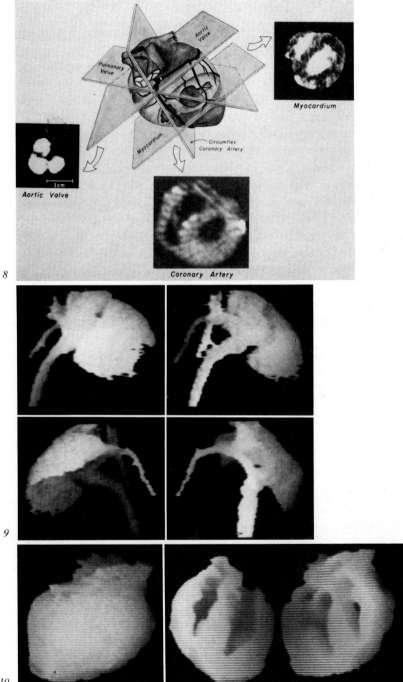

8

Aortic Valve

1cm

Pulmonary
Valve

Aortic
Valve

Myocardium

Myocardium

Circumflex
Coronary Artery

Coronary Artery

9

10

for different people and differs in the same patient in sequential studies. It must be almost impossible to predict accurately prior to a scan what these optimal locations and orientations should be. The critical issue here is that it is not much use making an accurate measurement if it is not in the right place. At this stage of development of the DSR, one of the greatest problems that we are facing is how to conveniently determine where to place the slice, within the volume scanned, needed to make an image for accurate measurement. There are several methods of analyzing the volume images [3, 4]. Two applications of one powerful method are illustrated in figures 9 and 10. In the former, the blood distribution in the right ventricular chamber is displayed. With this exact outline information, accurate estimates of any cardiac chamber's volume, regardless of shape, can be made. This capability eliminates the need to use the simplifying assumptions, such as ellipsoid shape of the heart chambers. Figure 10 illustrates the same technique applied to heart muscle. This display technique permits 'cutting' the heart open to look inside at the chambers and heart wall thicknesses. Indeed, by adding up all the volume occupied by the heart wall, heart weight can be estimated.

In summary, the pathologists over the last 100 years or more have developed quite well-defined techniques for looking at certain anatomic aspects of the heart. The DSR allows us to non-invasively mimic these techniques in analyzing the three-dimensional image data.

References

1 Ritman, E.L.; Kinsey, J.H.; Robb, R.A.; Gilbert, B.K.; Harris, L.D.; Wood, E.H.: Three-dimensional imaging of the heart, lungs, and circulation. Science *210:* 273–280 (1980).
2 Ritman, E.L.; Kinsey, J.H.; Robb, R.A.; Harris, L.D.; Gilbert, B.K.: Physics and technical considerations in the design of the DSR: a high temporal resolution volume scanner. Am.J.Roentg.*134:* 369–374 (1980).
3 Harris, L.D.; Robb, R.A.; Yuen, T.S.; Ritman, E.L.: The display and visualization of 3-D reconstructed anatomic morphology: experience with the thorax, heart, and coronary vasculature of dogs. J.Comput.assist.Tomogr. *3:* 439–446 (1979).
4 Herman, G.T.; Liu, H.K.: Display of three-dimensional information in computed tomography. J.Comput.assist.Tomogr.*1:* 155–160 (1977).
5 Chevalier, P.A.; Wood, E.H.; Robb, R.A., and Ritman, E.L.: Synchronous volumetric computed tomography for quantitative studies of structural and functional dynamics of the respiratory system. In: Mathys, H., et al.: Prog.Resp.Res., vol.11, pp.1–32 (Karger, Basel 1979).

6   Ritman, E.L.; Robb, R.A.; Johnson, S.A.; Chevalier, P.A.; Gilbert, B.K.; Green-
    leaf, J.F.; Sturm, R.E., and Wood, E.H.: Quantitative imaging of the structure and
    function of the heart, lungs, and circulation.Mayo Clin.Proc.*53:* 3–11 (1978).
7   Robb, R.A.; Ritman, E.L.: High-speed synchronous volume computed tomography
    of the heart. Radiology *133:* 655–661 (1979).
8   Ruegsegger, P.E.; Ritman, E.L., and Wood, E.H.: Performance of a cylindrical
    CT scanning system for dynamic studies of the heart and lungs. Proc. San Diego
    Biomedical Symp., vol.16, pp.143–157 (1977).
9   Sinak, L.J.; Ritman, E.L.: Computerized transmission tomography of the heart
    and great vessels – experimental evaluation and clinical application (in press).
10 Robb, R.A.: X-Ray computed tomography: an engineering synthesis of multi-
    scientific principles. CRC crit.Rev.Bioengng 7 (4): 265–334 (1982).

Erik L.Ritman, MD, PhD, Head, Biodynamics Research Unit, Mayo Foundation,
Mayo Clinic, Mayo Graduate School of Medicine, Rochester, MN 55905 (USA)

Mod. Probl. Paediat., vol. 22, pp. 48–62 (Karger, Basel 1983)

Supero-Inferior Ventricle and Criss-Cross Atrioventricular Connections: An Analysis of the Myth and Mystery

Robert M. Freedom

The University of Toronto, Faculty of Medicine, The Hospital For Sick Children, Toronto, Ontario, Canada

Introduction

Some congenitally malformed biventricular hearts continue to fascinate and to provoke discussion. This is particularly true of hearts with supero-inferior ventricles or those hearts whose angiocardiography suggests the presence of so-called criss-cross atrioventricular connections [*Lev and Rowlatt*, 1961; *Anderson* et al., 1974, 1977; *Ando* et al., 1976; *Sato* et al., 1976; *Symons* et al., 1977]. There is the common misconception that hearts with supero-inferior ventricles have crossed atrioventricular connections and, conversely, that hearts with crossed atrioventricular connections have an unusual ventricular relationship. While these observations may be true, either can occur in isolation (fig. 1) [*Freedom* et al., 1978; *Van Praagh* et al., 1980a].

The major anatomic disturbance in hearts with supero-inferior ventricles is displacement of the ventricular mass about the horizontal plane (fig. 2). This is a post-septational rotational disturbance [*Franco-Vazquez* et al., 1973; *Kinsley* et al., 1974; *Guthaner* et al., 1976]. Implicit to supero-inferior ventricles is an unusual spatial orientation of the atrioventricular junction. But what is the mystery of criss-cross atrioventricular connections? Do the atrioventricular valves actually 'criss' or 'cross' in some mythical way? There is no doubt that most such hearts demonstrate both a strikingly abnormal ventricular relationship as well as a distorted spatial topography of the atrioventricular junctions. But reports from this institution [*Freedom* et al., 1978] and others [*Attie* et al., 1980; *Van Praagh* et al., 1980a] have indicated that the appearance of crossing atrioventricular connections is made even more dramatic by angiography, and that ventricular angio-

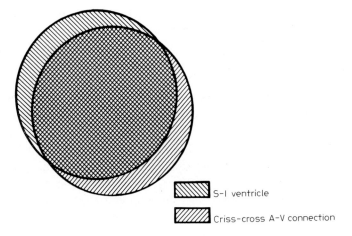

S-I ventricle

Criss-cross A-V connection

Fig.1. Venn diagramm showing that while supero-inferior ventricles or hearts with the angiocardiographic appearance of criss-cross atrioventricular connections can occur in isolation, they usually coexist.

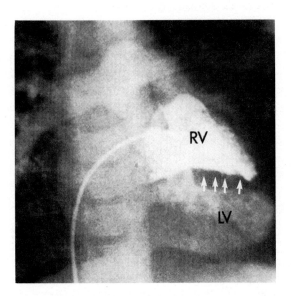

Fig.2. The angiocardiographic appearance of supero-inferior ventricles with the disposition of the ventricular mass about the horizontal plane. The morphologically right ventricle (RV) is the superiorly positioned ventricle, and the morphologically left ventricle (LV) is the inferior one. The horizontal ventricular septum is seen (white arrows).

cardiography contributes to this *pseudo-illusion*. In these hearts, the visual perception of an abnormal ventricular relationship as defined by angio-cardiography may not suggest the correct (or appropriate) type of atrio-ventricular connection, but rather may mislead [*Freedom* et al., 1978; *Attie* et al., 1980; *Van Praagh* et al., 1980a]. Thus, there are some hearts whose ventricular angiocardiographic appearance and relationship suggest a dis-cordant atrioventricular connection when, in fact, the connection is con-cordant – or vice versa.

But is the drama or pseudo-illusion of criss-crossing atrioventricular connections maintained by necropsy examination of a congenitally mal-formed heart whose angiographic appearance was that of supero-inferior ventricles with crossing atrioventricular connections? I think not! In the autopsy room, the prosector opens the morphological right atrium, visualizes the orifice of the right atrioventricular junction, probes the ventricular cavity with his finger via this orifice, and then opens into the ventricle following the flow of blood. The prosector may be aware of the unusual topography of the ventricles and their septum as well as the malorientation of the atrioventricular junction, but the nature of the atrioventricular junc-tion and its connection are easily defined (fig. 3).

What then is so curious about the angiographic appearance of these hearts? The answer rests in part on the angiographic criteria by which 'rightness' or 'leftness' is conferred to a ventricle. How does ventricular angiography permit assessment of the ventricular relationship? What is the role of atrial angiography? Fundamental to the understanding of these curious hearts is the realization that the internal organization of a ventricle, that ventricular relationships in space, and that the type of atrioventricular connection convey important, but different aspects of a congenitally mal-formed heart.

The Ventricular Relationship

The ventricular relationships as shown in figure 2 is clearly abnormal. The morphologically right ventricle is superior to the morphologically left ventricle. The ventricular septum is horizontal [*Kinsley* et al., 1974; *Guthaner* et al., 1976; *Waldhausen* et al., 1977; *Freedom* et al., 1978; *Zach* et al., 1978, 1980; *Attie* et al., 1980], and unlike the ventricular septum in the normal individual [*Ceballos* et al., 1981] it is best profiled angiographically in the frontal plane [*Guthaner* et al., 1976; *Freedom* et al., 1978, 1980; *Attie* et al.,

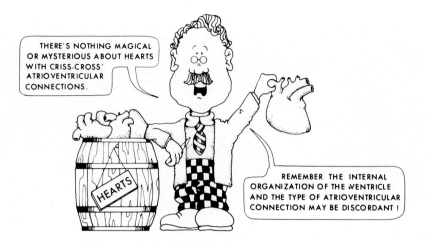

Fig. 3.

1980; *Van Praagh* et al., 1980a]. Most likely, the atrioventricular connection of this patient is concordant. However, selective right or left atriography filmed in frontal, lateral, left and right anterior oblique, or hepatoclavicular four-chamber projections are necessary to precisely define the character of the atrioventricular connections. The abnormal spatial relationship between the two ventricles of itself conveys no specific information about this connection [*Freedom* et al., 1978].

An inverted ventricular relationship (for the patient with atrial situs solitus) is suggested by left ventricular angiography in figure 4a. That is, the morphologically left ventricle appears to be to the right of the smaller, morphologically right ventricle. At least this is the perception given by the left ventriculogram. The spatial relationship (or our perception of the spatial relationship) between the two ventricles is consistent with a discordant type of atrioventricular connection. But what are we really seeing (fig. 4b–d)? Our attention is focused on the apical trabecular zone (and often the well-defined infundibular or outlet zone). But it is the character of the mural myocardium trabecular feature that confers 'rightness' or 'leftness' to the ventricle. Thus, in this patient (fig. 4a), the right-side of the angiographic silhouette is considered left-ventricular morphology ... and thus indicative of an inverted ventricular relationship. However, what the left ventriculogram in this patient does not demonstrate clearly is the inlet portion of the right ventricle. Thus, from figure 4a and b, one cannot be certain of the

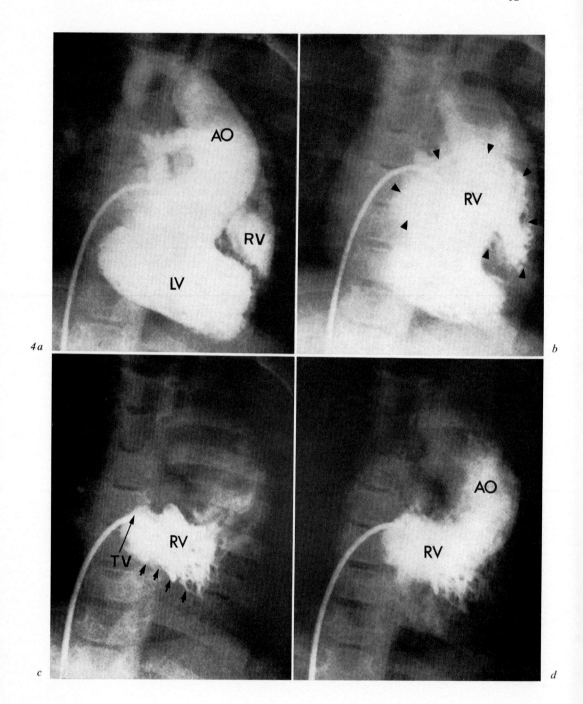

4a
b
c
d

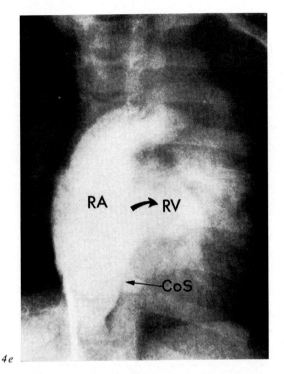

4e

Fig. 4. a Selective injection of contrast in the right-sided morphologically left ventricle (LV) suggests an inverted ventricular relationship with a left-sided morphologically and hypoplastic right ventricle (RV). *b* Another frame in the same sequence suggests the appearance of supero-inferior ventricles with the morphologically right ventricle (RV) superiorly positioned (outlined by arrowheads) and it appears better developed. *c, d* Selective injection in the superiorly positioned right ventricle (RV) via its inlet (TV) now demonstrates the character of this chamber in this patient with atrial situs solitus. *e* Selective right atriogram (RA) in frontal projection demonstrates concordant connection to superiorly positioned morphological right ventricle (RV). Note the horizontal ventricular septum (arrow) in *c*. CoS = Coronary sinus; AO = aorta.

internal organization of the right ventricle. Among most patients with the angiographic appearance of 'criss-cross', the atrium is connected to the ventricular inlet or the same side of the heart but there are exceptions (fig. 4e, 5) [*Weinberg* et al., 1980]. It is these exceptions that necessitate the distinction between the type of atrioventricular connection and the internal organization of the ventricle.

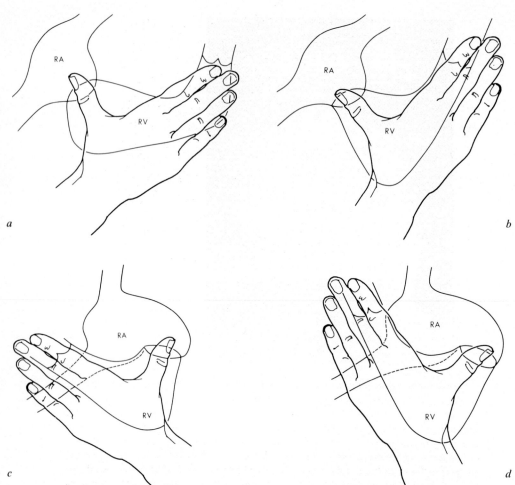

Fig. 5. Application of the *Van Praagh* et al. [1980a] hand-rule shown in diagrammatic form. *a* The normal relationship between the right atrium (RA) and right ventricle (RV). The internal organization of the morphological right ventricle conforms to the right-hand rule with the palmar surface of the right hand applied to the septal surface of the right ventricle, the right thumb notes the right atrioventricular junction; the base of thumb or wrist, the apical trabecular zone, and the fingertips, the outlet zone. *b* The right-hand pattern still applies when the morphological right ventricle is more horizontal than normal or frankly superior positioned. In *b* the atrioventricular junction is right-sided, while the outlet zone is clearly left-sided. *c, d* Clearly, despite a concordant-type of atrioventricular connection (an anatomic right atrium connected to the morphologic right ventricle), the internal organization of the morphologic right ventricle conforms to a left-hand pattern. Hearts with this very rare configuration *(c, d)* show clearly that the atrioventricular connection and internal organization of the right ventricle may be 'discordant'.

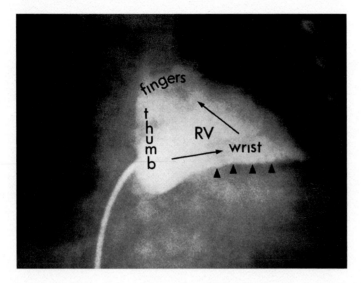

Fig.6. Application of the hand-rule to a patient with supero-inferior ventricles and superiorly positioned right ventricle (RV). The internal organization of this upstairs right ventricle conforms to a right-hand pattern of internal organization. Applying the palmar surface of the right hand to the septal surface of this heart necessitates and allows accurate characterization of the internal organization of the ventricle.

Internal Organization of the Ventricle

Van Praagh et al. (1980a] have defined the internal organization of the morphologically right ventricle as conforming to (1) a right hand pattern or (2) a left hand pattern. The application of the hand-rule necessitates that the palmar surface of the hand be placed on the septal surface of the morphological right ventricle, with the thumb identifying the inlet zone; the wrist, the apical trabecular zone; and the fingers, the infundibular or outlet zone (fig. 5, 6). In the individual with atrial situs solitus and a normal heart, it is the *right-hand pattern* that is characteristic of the morphologically right ventricle. The internal organization of the morphologically right ventricle conforms to the *left-hand pattern* in the individual with so-called atrial situs solitus and congenitally corrected transposition of the great arteries (atrioventricular and ventriculoarterial discordance).

Despite any unusual ventricular relationship, the concept of a right-hand or left-hand pattern of ventricular internal organization can be applied. This is particularly germane to supero-inferior ventricles or hearts with the angiographic appearance of criss-cross atrioventricular connections (fig. 6,

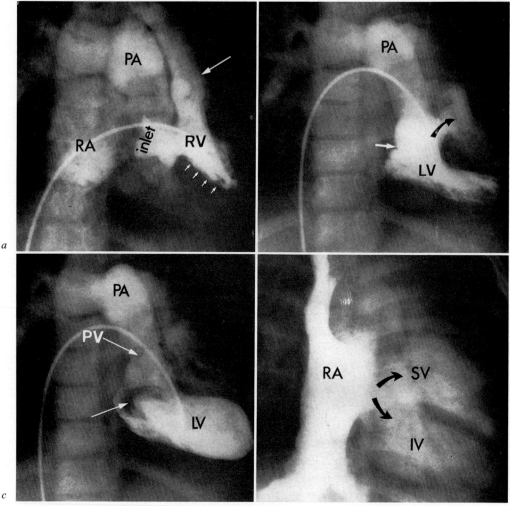

Fig. 7. Supero-inferior ventricles in a patient with right-sided straddling tricuspid valve. *a* Selective injection in morphologically right ventricle (RV) via a right-sided inlet. Both the pulmonary artery (PA) and the levo-positioned aorta (long white arrow) are opacified from this injection. The morphological right ventricle is somewhat small and the plane of the ventricular septum (small white arrow) is best visualized in the frontal plane. Reflux of contrast into the right-sided anatomic right atrium (RA) is evident. *b* Selective injection in the inferiorly positioned left ventricle (LV) presumed inlet to the left ventricle is noted (white arrow). *c* A slightly later frame in diastole shows the typical morphological appearance of a left ventricle (LV) with a non-opacified blood entering the left ventricle. Clearly, there is separation between the mitral inflow and the pulmonary valve (PV). *d* Selective right atriogram (RA) in frontal projection with opening of the right atrioventricular valve, there is simultaneous opacification of both ventricles, a superior ventricle (SV) and an inferiorly positioned one (LV).

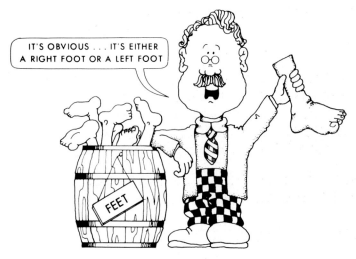

Fig.8.

7). The internal organization of a ventricle can best be defined angiographically by selective ventriculography, often in concert with selective atriography [*Attie* et al., 1980; *Freedom* et al., 1978, 1980; *Van Praagh* et al., 1980a]. In the individual with atrial situs solitus and concordant atrioventricular connections with rare exception the internal organization of the morphological right ventricle conforms to the right-hand pattern (fig. 5a, b). Similarly, the right ventricular organization of the individual with atrial situs solitus and discordant atrioventricular connections usually conforms to the left-hand pattern. *Weinberg* et al. [1980] have reported three hearts where the internal organization of the morphologically right ventricle was not predictive of the type of atrioventricular connection (fig. 5c, d). Thus, these hearts have a 'rosetta-stone' function. They force upon us the reality that the type of atrioventricular connection (concordant or discordant) does not invariably imply the internal organization of the morphological right ventricle, and that the ventricular relationship per se is another individual variable. Thus, if one could have a container filled with left feet or right feet, it is imminently clear as each foot is taken from the container whether it is a right foot or left foot. One can immediately appreciate the 'connection', but this is not true for the cardiac ventricle (fig. 3, 8). Hearts of the type mentioned above do not challenge the segmental approach [*Van Praagh*, 1972; *Tynan* et al., 1979] to cardiac diagnosis. Rather, they serve as prime advertisements for this approach and its application.

Application of a Segmental Approach to Hearts with Supero-Inferior Ventricles and the Angiocardiographic Appearance of Crossed Atrioventricular Connections.

One can define these hearts in terms of heart position, atrial situs, ventricular relationship, internal organization of the ventricle, atrioventricular connection, ventriculoarterial connection, great artery relationship, and associated malformations. This type of segmental analysis of the 50 some patients recorded in the literature yields the following profile.

Heart Position. Laevocardia was identified in about 75%, mesocardia in 10%, and dextrocardia in 15%.

Atrial Situs. Visceroatrial situs solitus is found in 88–90% of patients, atrial situs inversus (usually with dextrocardia) in 8–10%, right or left atrial isomerism is very uncommon.

Ventricular Relationship. The vast majority of patients exhibited a supero-inferior ventricular relationship with the morphologically right ventricle superior to the inferior positioned left ventricle (fig. 2–4, 6, 7).

Internal Organization of the Morphological Right Ventricle. Excluding the 3 patients reported by *Weinberg* et al. [1980], in the patient with atrial situs solitus, a concordant atrioventricular connection implied a right-hand pattern of organization, and a discordant connection would be consistent with a left-hand pattern (figs. 4, 5).

Atrioventricular Connection. About 60% reported patients were found to have concordant atrioventricular connections, about 20% discordant, and in the remainder one atrioventricular valve straddled the ventricular septum (fig. 7) [*Danielson* et al., 1979; *Becker* et al., 1980; *Freedom* et al., 1978, 1980; *Van Praagh* et al., 1980a].

Type of Infundibulum. Van Praagh et al. [1980b] have defined four types of infundibula: (1) subpulmonary; (2) subaortic; (3) bilaterally present infundibula; and (4) bilaterally deficient. Bilaterally deficient infundibula were not seen in these patients, and a solitary subpulmonary infundibulum was only occasionally seen (i.e. less than 10%). Most of the patients had either bilateral muscular subarterial infundibula or a subaortic infundibulum (fig. 7, 9).

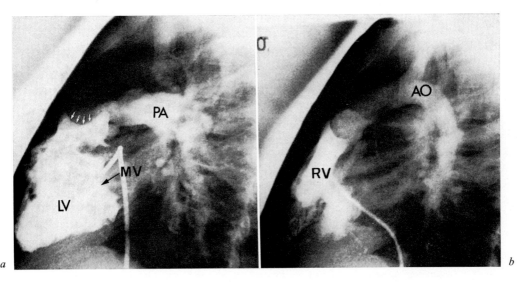

Fig. 9. Although any type of ventriculoarterial connection is possible, discordant or double-outlet right ventricle are the most commonly observed. *a* Lateral injection in small right ventricle (RV) shows the discordantly connected aorta (AO); *b* the lateral left ventriculogram (LV) via the mitral valve (MV) shows the pulmonary artery (PA) originating from a superior positioned ventricle. Another semilunar valve (white arrows) is evident.

Ventriculoarterial Connection. Four types of ventriculoarterial connections have been identified in these patients. A single outlet aorta (probably originating from the morphological left ventricle) was identified in 1 patient, and normal ventriculoarterial connection was noted in less than 10 % of the reported else [*Sato* et al., 1978; *Van Praagh* et al., 1980a]. Double-outlet from the anatomic right ventricle was observed in about 25 % [*Van Praagh* et al., 1980a], and in the majority, the ventriculoarterial connection was discordant or that of transposition (fig. 7, 9).

Great Artery Relationships. The relative position of the two semilunar valves are seldom normal. The aortic valve was identified as either right-anterior or right side-by-side of the pulmonary valve in about half of the reported patients and, in the remainder, the aortic valve is left-anterior or left-side by side (fig. 1, 7). One of the consistent features of these types of hearts is that the position of the aortic valve is not predictive of the atrioventricular connection [*Freedom* et al., 1974, 1978; *Otero Coto* et al., 1978; *Van Praagh* et al., 1980a].

Associated Malformations

Ventricular Hypoplasia. Hypoplasia of the anatomic right ventricle is common in these hearts, and the hypoplasia affects the right ventricular inlet and apical trabecular zones [*Anderson* et al., 1974; *Freedom* et al., 1978, 1980; *Attie* et al., 1980; *Van Praagh* et al., 1980a]. This is in contrast to the often left-sided and well-expanded right ventricular subarterial infundibulum that usually supports the aorta or both great arteries (fig 1, 5, 7).

Ventricular Septal Defect. All patients had ventricular septal defects. Because many of the patients have not undergone necropsy examination, it is difficult to precisely characterize the position of the ventricular septal defect. Among the patients with double-outlet right ventricle, the ventricular septal defect was often large, subpulmonary, and located between the limbs of the trabecula septomarginalis [*Anderson* et al., 1974; *Freedom* et al., 1978, 1980; *Milo* et al., 1979; *Van Praagh* et al., 1980a]. The patients with discordant atrioventricular connections tended to have large posterior ventricular septal defects of the AV defect type, and these defects were often confluent with defects of the infundibular septum which resulted from malalignment. Less common was the isolated membranous ventricular septal defect or the isolated defect of the infundibular septum.

Pulmonary Outflow Tract Obstruction. Pulmonary outflow tract obstruction is common, occurring in about half of the reported patients. As one might anticipate, potentially multiple mechanisms could be responsible for subpulmonary obstruction. The most frequent mechanism is a poorly expanded subpulmonary infundibulum, but atrioventricular valve tissue may also participate [*Van Praagh* et al., 1980a]. The pulmonary valve may also be stenotic, but this does not occur in this setting in isolation. Pulmonary atresia has been identified in 2 patients [*Anderson* et al., 1974; *Freedom* et al., 1978].

Aortic Outflow Tract Obstruction. Subaortic stenosis and/or coarctation of the aorta was observed in about 20 % of the patients. Because the transposed aorta originates above a hypoplastic right ventricle, it is not surprising that an obstructive anomaly of the aortic arch might be present.

Miscellaneous Anomalies. Juxtaposition of the atrial appendages, usually left juxtaposition of the right atrial appendage, was found in about 10 % of the patients [*Wagner* et al., 1970; *Freedom* et al., 1978; *Otero Coto* et al., 1979]. Cor triatriatum was observed in 1 patient.

References

Anderson, K.R.; Lie, J.T.; Sieg, D.; Hagler, D.J.; Ritter, D.G.; Davis, G.D.: A criss-cross heart. Detailed anatomic description and discussion of morphogenesis. Mayo Clin.Proc.*52:* 569 (1977).

Anderson, R.H.; Shinebourne, E.A.; Gerlis, L.M.: Criss-cross atrioventricular relationships producing paradoxical atrioventricular concordance or discordance. Their significance to nomenclature of congenital heart disease. Circulation *50:* 176 (1974).

Ando, M.; Takao, A.; Nihmura, I.; Mori, K.: Crossing atrioventricular valves. Clinical study of 8 cases. Circulation *53/54:* suppl. II, p.90 (1976).

Attie, F.; Munoz-Castellanos, L.; Ovseyevitz, J.; Flores-Delgado, I.; Testelli, M.R.; Buendia, A.; Kuri, J.; Molina,B.: Crossed atrioventricular connections. Am.Heart J. *99:* 163 (1980).

Becker, A.E.; Yen Ho, S.; Caruso, G.; Milo, S.; Anderson, R.H.: Straddling right atrioventricular valves in atrioventricular discordance. Circulation *61:* 1133 (1980).

Ceballos, R.; Soto, B.; Bargeron, L.M., jr.: Angiographic anatomy of the normal heart through axial angiography. Circulation *64:* 351 (1981).

Danielson, G.D.; Tabry, I.F.; Ritter, D.G.; Fulton, R.E.: Surgical repair of criss-cross heart with straddling atrioventricular valve. J.thorac.cardiovasc.Surg.*77:* 847 (1979).

Franco-Vazquez, J.S.; Perez-Trevino, C.; Gaxiola, A.: Corrected transposition of the great arteries with extreme counter-clockwise torsion of the heart. Acta cardiol. *28:* 636 (1973).

Freedom, R.M.; Culham, G.; Rowe, R.D.: The criss-cross and superoinferior ventricular heart: an angiocardiographic study. Am.J.Cardiol*42:* 620 (1978).

Freedom, R.M.; Duncan, W.J.; Rowe, R.D.: The straddling and overriding atrioventricular valve: morphological and diagnostic features; in Gallucci, Bini, Thiene, Selected topics in cardiac surgery (Patron Editore Bologna, Bologna 1980).

Freedom, R.M.; Harrington, D.P.; White, R.I., Jr.: The differential diagnosis of levotransposed or malposed aorta. An angiocardiographic study. Circulation *50:* 1040 (1974).

Guthaner, D.; Higgins, C.B.; Silverman, J.F.; Hayden, W.G.; Wexler, L.: An unusual form of the transposition complex. Uncorrected levo-transposition with horizontal ventricular septum: report of two cases. Circulation *53:* 190 (1976).

Kinsley, R.H.; McGoon, D.C.; Danielson, G.K.: Corrected transposition of the great arteries. Associated ventricular rotation. Circulation *49:* 574 (1974).

Lev, M.; Rowlatt, U.F.: The pathologic anatomy of mixed levocardia. A review of thirteen cases of atrial or ventricular inversion with or without corrected transposition. Am.J.Cardiol.*8:* 216 (1961).

Milo, S.; Yen Ho, S.; Macartney, F.J.; Wilkinson, J.L.; Becker, A.E.; Wenick, A.C.G.; Gittenberger-D Groot, A.C.; Anderson, R.H.: Straddling and overriding atrioventricular valves: morphology and classification. Am.J.Cardiol.*44:* 1122 (1979).

Otero Coto, E.; Quero Jimenez, M.; Cabrera, A.; Deverall, P.B.; Caffarena, J.M.: Aortic levopositions without ventricular inversion. Eur.J.Cardiol. *8:* 523 (1978).

Otero Coto, E.; Wilkinson, J.L.; Dickinson, D.F.; Rufilanchas, J.J.; Marques, J.: Gross distorsion of atrioventricular and ventriculo-arterial relations associated with left juxtaposition of atrial appendages. Bizarre form of atrioventricular criss-cross. Br. Heart J. *41:* 486 (1979).

Sato, T.; Kano, I.; Fukuda, M.; Yoshida, Y.; Sasaki, T.; Hoshino, H.: Angiocardiographic findings and morphogenesis of criss-cross heart with situs solitus, concordant atrioventricular relationships and *L*-transposition. Tohoku J.exp.Med. *119:* 377 (1976).

Sato, K.; Ohara, S.; Tsukaguchi, I.; Yasui, K.; Nakada, T.; Tamai, M.; Kobayashi, Y.; Kozuka, T.: A criss-cross heart with concordant atrioventriculo-arterial connections. Report of a case. Circulation *57:* 396 (1978).

Symons, J.C.; Shinebourne, E.A.; Joseph, M.C.; Lincoln, C.; Ho, Y.; Anderson, R.H.: Criss-cross heart with congenitally corrected transposition: report of a case with *d*-transposed aorta and ventricular preexcitation. Eur.J.Cardiol. *5:* 493 (1977).

Tynan, M.J.; Becker, A.E.; Macartney, F.J.; Quero-Jimenez, M.; Shinebourne, E.A.; Anderson, R.H.: Nomenclature and classification of congenital heart disease. Br. Heart J. *41:* 544 (1979).

Van Praagh, R.: The segmental approach to diagnosis in congenital heart disease. Birth defects: original article series (Williams & Wilkins, Baltimore 1972).

Van Praagh, S.; LaCorte, M.; Fellows, K.E.; Bossina, K.; Buach, H.J.; Keck, E.W.; Weinberg, P.M.; Van Praagh, R.: Supero-inferior ventricles: anatomic and angiocardiographic findings in ten postmortem cases; in Van Praagh, Takao, Etiology and morphogenesis of congenital heart disease (Futura Publishing, New York 1980a).

Van Praagh, R.; Layton, W.M.; Van Praagh, S.: The morphogenesis of normal and abnormal relationships between the great arteries and the ventricles: pathologic and experimental data; in Van Praagh, Takao, Etiology and morphogenesis of congenital heart disease (Futura Publishing, New York 1980b).

Wagner, H.R.; Alday, L.E.; Vlad, P.: Juxtaposition of the atrial appendages. A report of six necropsied cases. Circulation *42:* 157 (1970).

Waldhausen, J.A.; Pierce, W.S.; Whitman, V.: Horizontal interventricular septum in congenital heart disease: surgical consideration. Ann.thor.Surg. *23:* 271 (1977).

Weinberg, P.M.; Van Praagh, R.; Wagner, H.R.; Cuaso, C.C.: New form of criss-cross atrioventricular relation: an expanded view of the meaning of *D* and *L*-loops. Wld Congr. Paediatric Cardiology, London 1980, p.319.

Zach, M.; Beitzke, A.; Gypser, G.; Hofler, H.: Die Transposition der grossen Gefässe mit horizontalem interventrikularem Septum. Herz *3:* 133 (1978).

Zach, M.; Singer, M.; Lojer, H.; Hagel, K.J.: The horizontal interventricular septum: three cases with different ventriculoarterial connections. Eur.J.Cardiol. *11:* 269 (1980).

Robert M.Freedom, MD, Professor of Paediatrics and Pathology, The University of Toronto, Faculty of Medicine, Senior Staff Physician, The Hospital for Sick Children, Toronto, Ont. (Canada)

Mod. Probl. Paediat., vol. 22, pp. 63–67 (Karger, Basel 1983)

Surgical Treatment of Congenital Cardiac Malformations in Children under 2 Years of Age

A. Frigiola, L. Menicanti, L. Bedogni, G. P. Belloli

Division of Pediatric Surgery, Cardiothoracic Unit, Regional Hospital, Vicenza, Italy

In recent years there has been an increasing interest towards early correction of congenital heart disease in young patients. This work considers the results obtained by the Cardiothoracic Pediatric Surgery Unit of the Vicenza Regional Hospital. In almost 5 years of cardiosurgical activity, 261 children under the age of 2 years have been operated in our institution. Of these, 159 had closed heart surgery and 102 had open heart surgery (table I).

Palliative Surgery

The palliative interventions carried out in children under the age of 2 years and the relative pathology are listed in table II. In the group with decreased pulmonary flow, in general we perform a Blalock-Taussig shunt or we use a Gore-Tex tubular prosthesis. The choice is conditioned by the type of malformation and the anatomic situation. In the presence of a complex malformation in which complete correction is foreseen after 4–5 years, we prefer to apply a Gore-Tex prosthesis on the side opposite to the aortic arch, enabling us to carry out a Blalock-Taussig shunt at a later date. We use, instead, the Gore-Tex prosthesis independently of the malformation, when we consider that the anatomic situation is unfavorable and there is a serious doubt that the systemic-pulmonary anastomosis may not be functioning completely. We prefer not to carry out the Waterston shunt because we consider, according to many other autors, that such a type of shunt may give some complications, such as cardiac failure in the postoperative period, pulmonary hypertension or obstructive kinking of the pulmonary artery.

Table I. Division of Pediatric Surgery, Cardiothoracic Unit, Vicenza: summary of cardiac procedure under age 2 years

	Number of patients	Cardiac mortality (%)
Closed heart operation	159	12 (11.7)
Open heart operation	102	16 (15.7)
Total	261	28 (10.7)

Table II. Division of Pediatric Surgery, Cardiothoracic Unit, Vicenza: palliative surgical operations under age 2 years

Operation	Number of patients	Deaths cardiac (%)	non-cardiac (%)
Pulmonary-systemic shunt	64	6 (9.3)	
Pulmonary artery banding	22	1 (4.5)	1 (4.5)
Blalock-Hanlon	11	1 (9.0)	
Others	4	1 (25.0)	
Total	101	9 (8.9)	1 (0.9)

Banding of the pulmonary artery has been carried out on 22 infants with ventricular septal defect and once in a patient with a complete atrioventricular canal, who died of a sudden cardiac arrest on the tenth postoperative day. We carried out the banding with a Teflon ribbon according to Trusler's data. We obtained good results with banding in the cases with cardiac failure and increased pulmonary flow. In a patient with a large muscular defect with intractable cardiac failure, the defect closed spontaneously 20 months after banding procedure. In the CAVC if possible, we avoid the pulmonary artery banding, because of the high mortality rate, and prefer therefore corrective surgery even during the first months of life. We carried out 11 Blalock-Hanlon procedures. 10 cases were simple transposition of the great arteries (TGA), and 1 a case of TGA and ventricular septal defect (VSD). Our present policy is to limit such surgical procedure, preferring at the beginning the balloon septostomy followed by 'physiologic' correction after the first 3 months of life.

Corrective Surgery

Closed Heart Surgery. Our results are listed in table III. We have operated on 27 patients with aortic coarctation, of which 5 had serious hypoplasia of the aortic arch. In only 3 cases with associated VSD and pulmonary hypertension we carried out a pulmonary artery banding. In 4 cases we utilized a subclavian flap technique. In the remaining patients end-to-end anastomosis was performed. We have had 4 deaths; three occurred because they had associated cardiac malformations, the fourth was caused by severe Salmonella sepsis. In the patent ductus arteriosus group, 26 cases, no deaths have occurred. In 2 cases of pulmonary valvular stenosis with good right ventricle we carried out a transpulmonary valvulotomy.

Open Heart Surgery. Extracorporeal circulation was employed in all the cases. For the simple defects we used mild hypothermia (28–30 °C) while for the complex cases we used a variable temperature from 28 to 18 °C according to the type of malformation and the weight of the child. Deep hypothermia with cardiocirculatory arrest was used in all the cases of TGA, total anomalous pulmonary venous return (TAPVR) and pulmonary stenosis in children weighing less than 3 kg. Deep hypothermia was induced within a few cases at the beginning of our activity. Since then we have used the core-cooling deep hypothermia. In all the cases of aortic cross-clamping we used cardioplegia. Our results are listed in tables IV and V.

The indication of the intervention is given by serious cardiac failure uncontrollable by medical therapy or by a progressive increasing of the pulmonary resistances. All the VSD were closed by transatrial approach and the patch was sewed by detached stitches. Of the 4 deaths, 2 occurred in children that were less than 3 months old; we actually prefer to carry out, at this age, pulmonary artery banding.

In the TGA, we use the Senning technique which we carried out generally after the first 3 months of life. Of the 31 operated cases, the 2 deaths occurred in 2 children respectively 2 and 45 days old. In the severe forms of pulmonary stenosis, our present policy is the complete correction in ECC associated or not to deep hypothermia in the first few months of life.

In addition to valvulotomy we usually patch the infundibulum with the pericardium. The only death occurred in an infant on the twelfth day of the postoperative period probably because of an infundibular spasm. In this case an infundibular patch was not used.

Table III. Division of Pediatric Surgery, Cardiothoracic Unit, Vicenza: closed cardiac operations under age 2 years

Malformation	Number of patients	Deaths	
		cardiac (%)	non-cardiac (%)
Aortic coarctation	27	3 (11.1)	1 (3.7)
Patent ductus arteriosus	26	–	
Pulmonary artery stenosis	2	–	
Others	3	–	
Total	58	3 (5.1)	1 (1.7)

Table IV. Division of Pediatric Surgery, Cardiothoracic Unit, Vicenza: open cardiac operations under age 2 years

Malformation	Number of patients	Deaths	
		cardiac (%)	non-cardiac (%)
Ventricular septal defect	39	4 (10.2)	1 (2.5)
Transposition of the great arteries	31	2 (6.4)	
Pulmonary artery stenosis	9	1 (11.1)	
Total anomalous pulmonary venous return	5	2 (40.0)	
Complete atrioventricular canal	7	2 (28.5)	1 (14.2)
Tetralogy of Fallot	6	2 (33.3)	
Double outlet right ventricle	2	1 (50)	
Others	3	2 (66.6)	
Total	102	16 (15.6)	2 (1.9)

Table V. Division of Pediatric Surgery, Cardiothoracic Unit, Vicenza: open heart surgery under age 2 years

Age, months	Number of patients	Deaths	
		cardiac (%)	non-cardiac (%)
< 6	36	10 (27.7)	1 (2.7)
6–12	20	–	–
12–24	46	6 (13.0)	1 (2.1)
Total	102	16 (15.6)	2 (1.9)

6 patients with tetralogy of Fallot were corrected in the first few months of life; 2 deaths have been recorded. Actually, we follow the more recent indications of the University of Alabama, and therefore we avoid complete correction of children under the age of 2 years, with the exception of those patients with favorable anatomy and a body surface area of more than 0.35 m². In the majority of cases we prefer however to perform a systemic-pulmonary shunt and to postpone the total correction until the third or fourth year of life. In effect, in our series of total correction for tetralogy of Fallot above the age of 3 years we did not have any deaths; neither did we have mortality caused by cardiac failure in the cases of Fallot palliated by Blalock-Taussig or PTFE shunts.

There have been 7 CAVC corrections with 2 deaths, 1 of which for insufficiency of the mitral valve on the fourth postoperative day and the second for low cardiac output syndrome.

Of the 5 cases of TAPVR, there were 3 supradiaphragmatic, 1 in coronary sinus, and 1 was infradiaphragmatic. The 2 deaths occurred in new-born children, respectively 4- and 6-day-old with serious pulmonary hypertension. In both cases there remained an atrial septal defect.

This series is limited, but we think that these results, obtained with a selective and rational choice between palliation and complete surgical repair, are very encouraging.

Alessandro Frigiola, MD, Divisione di Chirurgia Pediatrica, Sezione di cardio-chirurgia, Ospedale Generale Regionale, I-36100 Vicenza (Italy)

Mod. Probl. Paediat., vol. 22, pp. 68–69 (Karger, Basel 1983)

Management of Severe Coarctation of the Aorta in the First Month of Life

Garrick I. Fiddler, Ranjit R. Chatrath, Duncan R. Walker

Regional Paediatric Cardiology Centre, Killingbeck Hospital, Leeds, England

The neonate with severe aortic coarctation may present a difficult problem in terms of investigation and management. Between 1978 and 1981 we treated 36 such neonates. There were 19 males and 17 females: mean age was 12 days (1–28 days), mean weight was 3.1 kg (1.8–4.5 kg).

The majority of patients (32/36) were in heart failure. 8 patients had oliguria and 3 were anuric. Associated defects were demonstrated at angiography in 23 of the patients. This excludes a ductus arteriosus which was present in all the patients (table I).

After initial assessment and resuscitation where necessary, all the patients underwent immediate surgery. A subclavian flap aortoplasty was performed in 34 patients and a Gore-Tex patch was used in 2 patients (table II). Dopamine (2–8 μg/kg/min) was used in the perioperative period in 21 patients who were ill with heart failure and acidosis including the 11 with pre-operative renal dysfunction. Only 1 patient of the 18 with an associated ventricular septal defect (VSD) required closure of the defect at the age of 8 months.

Operative mortality was 5.5 % (2 patients). There were 3 late deaths in patients with complex associated malformations – 1 involving the gastro-intestinal system and 2 with complex congenital cardiac defects. 3 patients (8 %) required revision of the aortoplasy using a Gore-Tex patch 3–18 months later. All the other patients are well.

We conclude that with a combination of vigorous resuscitation including dopamine infusion, when necessary, neonatal coarctation can be safely managed with a low operative mortality. In our experience the group of coarctation patients with an associated VSD do not require pulmonary artery banding in the neonatal period. With careful ventilatory management

Table I. Symptoms and associated defects in 36 neonates with coarctation of the aorta

	Patients (%)
Heart failure	32 (89)
Renal dysfunction	11 (30)
Associated defects	23 (63)
VSD	18
Aortic stenosis	4
Complex	4

Table II. Operations and management of the neonate with coarctation of the aorta

	Patients
Subclavian flap aortoplasty	34
Gore-Tex patch	2
Dopamine in the peri-operative period	21
VSD repair	1 (at age 8 months)

in the peri-operative period they can be extubated within a few days of surgery. Only 1 of the 18 VSD patients later required corrective surgery. The VSD in the other patients is small or diminishing in size as judged on clinical evidence with supporting echocardiographic or haemodynamic data.

Garrick I. Fiddler, Regional Paediatric Cardiology Centre, Killingbeck Hospital, York Road, Leeds LS14 6UQ (England)

Mod. Probl. Paediat., vol. 22, pp. 70–75 (Karger, Basel 1983)

Palliative Surgery in Tricuspid Atresia: Early and Late Results

G. A. Trusler

Department of Surgery, University of Toronto and the Hospital for Sick Children, Toronto, Ontario, Canada

The development of the Fontan operation brought a new dimension to the treatment of tricuspid atresia and made accurate determination of the intracardiac anatomy of major importance [2]. Similarly, the anatomy of the great vessels, the size of the pulmonary arteries, the resistance in the pulmonary vascular bed and the function of the left ventricle are vital. The palliative procedures, used in early life, must be tailored not only to provide long-term palliation, but to prepare and maintain the cardiovascular system. Therefore, shunts and other procedures must not only provide adequate oxygen saturation, but must maintain the patency and size of the pulmonary arteries, and, at the same time, avoid increased pulmonary vascular resistance.

Clinical Experience

To outline the long-term results, I will review our experience from 1947 to 1980. In that 33-year period, 159 infants and children with tricuspid atresia were treated by one or more operations.

Of those with known anatomy, 81 % had normally related great arteries and approximately two thirds or 62 % were type 1B which is perhaps the most suitable type for a Fontan procedure since there is a small right ventricular chamber and outflow tract which may be used in the repair (table I).

First Palliative Operation

Although there were some others with initially increased pulmonary blood flow, only 12 of the 159 children had pulmonary artery banding.

Table I. Anatomic classification of tricuspid atresia

Type	I	II (D-TGA)	III (L-TGA)
A Pulmonary atresia	18	4	3
B Pulmonary stenosis	94 (62%)	11	2
C No pulmonary stenosis	10	7	1
	122 (81%)	22	6

Group IV, 1; unknown, 8.
TGA = Transposition of the great arteries.

6 of the 8 survivors have since had shunt procedures, 2 a Glenn anastomosis and 4 a Blalock-Taussig shunt for further palliation. Two required other operations, one a creation of aortopulmonary window for restrictive bulbo-ventricular foramen, and another, a left ventricular aortic conduit for severe aortic stenosis. 1 boy with a restrictive bulboventricular foramen had both an arterial repair of his transposed great arteries and a Fontan repair.

Of the other 147 patients, 10 had a variety of first operations such as enlargement of ventricular septal defect and other desperate procedures some 20–30 years ago (table II, III). These and the bandings (22 patients) are included in the miscellaneous category. The other 137 children were palliated with shunts as their first operation. As expected, the mortality for the shunt is significantly high in the first 6 months of life. Just over half of the infants required operation at this time. Originally, we preferred the Potts anastomosis in this age group since it was the easiest and most reliable shunt to construct in a tiny infant. While the mortality was high in early years, it was much lower in the past 15 years.

In infants and children over 6 months of age, the Blalock anastomosis was most useful with a fairly low risk particularly recently. At one time, we were enthusiastic about the Glenn anastomosis as a primary shunt operation. It gave excellent early results with a very low mortality. However, it is more appropriate as a second shunt and, in recent years, it is seldom used as we observe the long-term results of both the Fontan and Glenn operations.

Subsequent Palliative Operation

60 or about half of the early survivors have required a second operation (table IV) 47 were shunt procedures and the Blalock-Taussig shunt was the most useful. The Potts shunt is not a satisfactory secondary procedure for it

Table II. Mortality with first operation < 6 months

	Number	Died
Potts	38	17
Blalock	18	6
Glenn	3	2
Waterston	6	2
Central	1	0
Miscellaneous	17	9
	83	36

Table III. Mortality with first operation > 6 months

	Number	Died
Potts	15	3
Blalock	33	3
Glenn	19	0
Waterston	3	1
Central	1	0
Miscellaneous	5	3
	76	10

Table IV. Second operation

	Number	Early death
Potts	9	1
Blalock	21	2
Glenn	14	1
Waterston	3	1
Miscellaneous	5	1
Fontan	8	2
	60	8

requires mobility of the pulmonary artery which is lost after the first shunt. The Glenn operation has been very useful and the only early death was a desperately ill infant in whom a large Waterston anastomosis was revised and a Glenn anastomosis carried out.

20 children have required a third operation (table V). Again, the Blalock and Glenn anastomoses were frequently used. Often by the time of the

Table V. Third Operation

	Number	Early death
Blalock	4	0
Glenn	2	1
Central	3	0
Axillary	3	0
Miscellaneous	1	1
Fontan	7	1
	20	3

third operation, both pleural spaces had been opened for the two previous shunts. At this time, a central shunt, often using a prosthetic graft is of value. In special circumstances where this cannot be done, the existing Glenn shunt can be enhanced significantly by the addition of an axillary arterio-venous fistula as described by *Glenn* et al. [3] and we did this in 3 patients.

1 patient who is now 23 years of age has had a total of five operations, the last two being a Glenn and a central aortopulmonary artery shunt.

Late Results

In addition to the early mortality, there have been 13 late deaths, 10 occurring between the first and second operations and 3 between the second and third operations. While 5 were of unknown cause, another 5 were likely related to the shunt or the primary heart problem. In this group, I include 2 with pulmonary infarcts, 1 with pulmonary hypertension following a long-term Blalock-Taussig shunt, 1 with sepsis and 1 with cardiac failure. At present, there are 89 patients potentially surviving. 75 were contacted in 1978: 10 were in the third decade of life and another 37 were between 10 and 20 years of age.

In those 75 patients, approximately one third were asymptomatic and two thirds had mild to moderate symptoms. 3 were severely restricted. There-fore, of the 159 patients entering this series over the 33-year period from 1947 to 1980, over one half still survive. It is interesting to note that 33 of these survivors have a Glenn anastomosis, 26 have a Potts and 43 have at least 1 Blalock-Taussig. 1 still has a Waterston, and 18 are surviving with a Fontan repair.

Discussion

The Blalock-Taussig anastomosis is, in general, the best shunt because it produces controlled pulmonary blood flow which seldom causes pulmonary vascular disease and it is easy to take down or ligate at subsequent repair. However, in our hands, the Blalock-Taussig anastomosis seldom grows and, therefore, depending on its size and the age at which it is constructed, the child will gradually outgrow the anastomosis.

When a Blalock anastomosis is constructed in an infant weighing less than 3 kg, there is a good chance that the child will grow out of the anastomosis within the next year or two. If the child is a potential candidate for a Fontan operation at, say, age 6–12 years, a second shunt will be needed to attain that age.

For a long time, the Potts shunt was our preference in tricuspid atresia for it is easily constructed in the first few months of life and produces a large flow. The anastomosis tends to grow with the child producing an adequate shunt for many years. If one contemplates a Glenn anastomosis as part of the future management, then the Potts has the further advantage that it is on the left side, leaving the right side for the Glenn. Unfortunately, it is difficult to control both the initial size and growth, and there is the very significant disadvantage that the Potts shunt tends to cause stenosis and distortion of the left pulmonary artery just as the Waterston shunt does with the right pulmonary artery. We were able to control the growth of the Potts anastomosis by leaving a loose ligature of silk as a band around the anastomosis [5]. However, with the development of the Fontan operation, the possibility of pulmonary artery stenosis was unacceptable and we abandoned the Potts shunt except in special cases.

The Glenn anastomosis is perhaps the safest shunt to create as long as it is not done in infants or in patients with increased pulmonary vascular resistance. It grows and provides good palliation at first, but it tends to fail about 6–8 years later as the patient outgrows the blood flow to the contralateral lung. With increasing hypoxemia there is a rising hematocrit which increases blood viscosity and slows the flow through the Glenn anastomosis.

On reviewing the hemoglobin and hematocrit estimations in our patients with Glenns, we found that about 6–8 years after the Glenn shunt is created, these become quite high [6]. When an arterial shunt is added, they return to a reasonable level and may remain there for many years, as long as 16 years in 1 patient. The combination of a Glenn shunt on the right plus an arterial shunt on the left has provided good long-term palliation with good arterial oxygen saturations and relatively little excessive load on the heart. In patients who, for some reason, are not candidates for a Fontan operation this is an alternative as long as the pulmonary vascular resistance in the right lung is low. None of our patients has developed an arteriovenous malformation in the lung, perhaps because most of the Glenn shunts were created at an older age than in some series.

With that background, our general management of tricuspid atresia at present is to maintain infants and children with arterial shunts until they are old enough for a Fontan repair.

In infants less than 6–12 months old, a left Blalock-Taussig shunt is preferred usually using a 5-mm Gortex graft as described by *deLeval* et al. [1]. The proximal arterioplasty described by *Laks and Castaneda* [4] has made the left Blalock-Taussig anastomosis more effective than before. Our preliminary experience, however, tends to favor the prosthetic graft.

In infants over 6–12 months of age, a right Blalock-Taussig anastomosis is done and should support the child until old enough for a Fontan repair. Certainly the advent of this operation has underlined the importance of properly selecting and executing the palliative operation. Time should bring further refinements to this scheme of management.

References

1   deLeval, M.R.; McKay, R.; Jones, M.; Stark, J.; Macartney, M.B.: Modified Blalock-Taussig shunt. J.thorac.cardiovasc.Surg.*81:* 112 (1981).
2   Fontan, F.; Baudet, E.: Surgical repair of tricuspid atresia. Thorax *26:* 240 (1971).
3   Glenn, W.W.L.; Fenn, J.E.: Axillary arteriovenous fistula. A means of supplementing blood flow through a cava-pulmonary artery shunt. Circulation *46:* 1013 (1972).
4   Laks, H.; Castaneda, A.R.- Subclavian arterioplasty for the ipsilateral Blalock-Taussig shunt. Ann.thorac.Surg.*19:* 319 (1975).
5   Trusler, G.A.; Kanzaki, Y.: Controlling the growth of aortopulmonary anastomoses in piglets. Archs Surg., Chicago *106:* 72 (1973).
6   Trusler, G.A.; Williams, W.G.: Long-term results of the Glenn procedure. Congenital Heart Disease: 229, 1979.

George A.Trusler, MD, Associate Professor of Surgery, University of Toronto School of Medicine, Head, Division of Cardiovascular Surgery, The Hospital for Sick Children, Toronto, Ont. (Canada)

Mod. Probl. Paediat., vol. 22, pp. 76–78 (Karger, Basel 1983)

Corrective Surgery for Tricuspid Atresia

Gordon K. Danielson

Department of Surgery, Mayo Foundation, Mayo Clinic, Mayo Graduate School of Medicine, Rochester, Minn., USA

Following the lead of Fontan, we employed cardiac valves in our first 2 patients with tricuspid atresia. In the first patient, operated upon in 1973, a heterograft valve was inserted in the right atrium above the superior vena cava and a nonvalved tube graft connected the right atrium to the rudimentary right ventricle. The second patient also had a heterograft valve placed in the right atrium, but a valved conduit connected the right atrial appendage to the pulmonary artery. We did not have fresh homografts available and, therefore, used the glutaraldehyde-preserved porcine valve which was available at that time.

We very quickly learned, however, that in the right atrium and in the atriopulmonary position, the glutaraldehyde valve has an accelerated rate of deterioration. Figure 1 shows a valve 4 years after placement in the right atrium. The leaflets have fused in the semi-open position and the valve is both stenotic and incompetent. Equally distressing, in this same patient, there were obstructive changes in the nonvalved Dacron tube graft connecting the right atrium to the right ventricle. The graft had a thick peel and extensive ulcerating calcification.

These degenerative changes resulted in our discontinuation of glutaraldehyde-preserved porcine valves and Dacron tube grafts. Whenever possible, we have employed some type of direct connection of right atrium to the right ventricle or pulmonary artery. We frequently use a modification of the Björk technique by creating a flap from the right atrial appendage to form the floor of the conduit. A generous piece of pericardium is then used to construct the sides and roof of the conduit. We have had no late stenoses following this procedure.

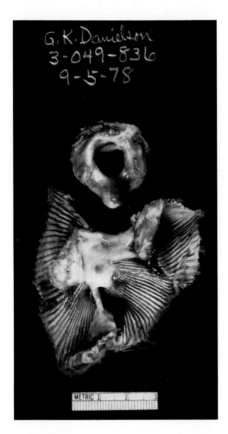

Fig. 1. Gluteraldehyde-preserved porcine valve and Dacron rube graft 4 years after operation. There are extensive degenerative changes in both. Direct anastomoses without valves are currently preferred.

From October 31, 1973, through July 31, 1981, 60 patients with tricuspid atresia have undergone the Fontan procedure at the Mayo Clinic. The ages ranged from 8 months to 33 years. 67 prior surgical procedures had been performed in 56 patients.

Dacron conduits were employed in 34 patients; 22 contained a glutaral-dehyde-preserved porcine valve and 12 were nonvalved. In the latter part of our experience, 26 patients have undergone direct anastomosis with or without pericardial patch augmentation. Concomitant cardiac procedures were performed in 5 patients. 2 patients had mitral valve replacement with a porcine xenograft, 1 had mitral anuloplasty, 1 underwent transplantation of the atrial septum for correction of pulmonary A–V fistulae in the right lower lobe secondary to a Glenn anastomosis, and the fifth patient had ligation of coronary artery fistulas. There were 8 deaths in the entire series of 60 patients for an overall mortality of 13.3%. Since 1976, 51 patients underwent operation with 5 deaths for a mortality of 9.8%.

There was a clear relationship of outcome to whether or not the patient met the ideal criteria for operation as outlined by Choussat and Fontan. 23 patients met all the criteria and there was only 1 death, a patient who fibrillated during postoperative cardiac catheterization (mortality 4.2%). 37 patients fell outside the ideal criteria in one or more categories. In this group there were 7 operative deaths for a mortality of 18.9%; however, most of the operative survivors have derived significant palliation from their procedure.

Gordon K. Danielson, MD, Department of Surgery, Mayo Foundation,
Mayo Clinic, Mayo Graduate School of Medicine, Rochester, MN 55905 (USA)

Mod. Probl. Paediat., vol. 22, pp. 79–82 (Karger, Basel 1983)

Complete Transposition of Great Arteries (TGA): Factors Influencing Survival after Balloon Atrial Septostomy

A. Agnetti[a], *R. Leanage*[b], *G. Graham*[b], *J. Taylor*[b], *F. Macartney*[b]

[a] Clinica Pediatrica, Università di Parma, Italy; [b] Hospital for Sick Children, London, England

The introduction of balloon atrial septostomy (BAS) in 1966 has dramatically altered the natural history of complete transposition of the great arteries (TGA). Before that era about 80 % of the patients died within the first 6 months of life, while now survival at the same period is about 80 % (fig. 1). However, in spite of BAS many children die, often in an unexpected and unexplained manner, before reaching definitive surgery. Is there any way of telling in advance which patients are going to die in this manner? Is it possible to be able to identify which are risk factors? In an attempt to solve this problem, a retrospective study of 144 patients with TGA was carried out. All had had BAS at the Hospital for Sick Children, London, for the period December 1966 to June 1978.

All findings thought important about clinical course and survival curve were considered. Those data were coded, and then analysed by a log rank test (a modification of the Mantel-Haenzel test) to identify which factors influence survival curve and their interactions. Finally the resulting factors were introduced into discriminant function analysis, in order to obtain prediction of survival at 6 months by survival probability tables. This prediction was correct in 76 % of the patients studied. From the previously described analytical methods, the statistically significant factors were: pulmonary artery systolic pressure; systemic arterial oxygen saturation; haemoglobin concentration; age at BAS; patent ductus arteriosus (PDA); ventricular septal defect (VSD); left ventricular outflow tract obstruction (LVOTO), and coarctation/aortic stenosis.

Pulmonary Artery Systolic Pressure. The pulmonary artery systolic pressure, taken at the second catheterization, was closely correlated with

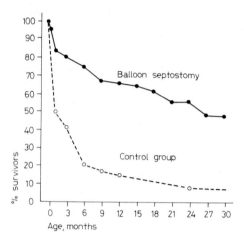

Fig.1. Survival of patients after BAS for TGA (excluding deaths at corrective surgery).

survival: at 8 months after BAS survival in patients with systolic pressure below 30 mm Hg was 94.0 ($\pm$2.9)%, in those with pressure between 30 and 50 mm Hg it was 92.3 ($\pm$7.4)%, in those with pressure between 50 and 70 mm Hg it was 60.0 ($\pm$21.9)%, and in those with pressure over 70 mm Hg it was 40.0 ($\pm$21.9)%.

Systemic Arterial Oxygen Saturation. The rise in systemic arterial oxygen saturation after BAS at the first catheterization was strongly predictive of survival, but the effect was non-linear. Patients did worst if there was a rise in saturation under 15%, and did better with either a higher rise, no change, or fall in oxygen saturation. While oxygen arterial and venous systemic saturation at the second catheterization, taken alone, had an effect on survival of borderline statistical significance, but adjustment for haemoglobin concentration greatly strengthened this relation, at 9 months of age survival was 74.6 ($\pm$8.4)% for patients with oxygen content inferior to 12 vol% and 92.9 ($\pm$6,9)% for patients with oxygen content over 12 vol%.

Haemoglobin Concentration. The lower the plasma haemoglobin concentration, the poorer the survival. This fact applied both at the time of BAS and at the second cardiac catheterization, routinely carried out between 4 and 6 months of life. The effect was particularly marked in patients with haemoglobin below 13.5 g/100 ml, in which survival at 5 months after BAS was 47.0 ($\pm$9.8)%, as opposed to 70.0 ($\pm$6.8)% for haemoglobin between 13.5 and 15 g/100 ml, and to 84.0 ($\pm$5.9)% for haemoglobin between 15.5 and 18 g/100 ml and to 78.7 ($\pm$9.6)% for haemoglobin over 18 g/100 ml.

Age at Balloon Atrial Septostomy. Patients who underwent BAS during the first week of life had at 6 months a survival of 71.6 ($\pm$5.4)%, patients who underwent BAS between 1 week and 4 weeks, had a survival of 39.3 ($\pm$9.6)%, while those with BAS after the first month of life had a survival of 50.2 ($\pm$11.0)%. We therefore interpret these findings as indicating that the older patients had relatively little need for septostomy, whereas the intermediate group needed septostomy, but they had it too late to be really effective.

Patent Ductus Arteriosus. Presence of PDA (or small PDA) always had a statistically significant negative effect on survival. For large non-ligated PDA it was deleterious: no patients of this group survived more than 5 days. At 1 year survival was 74.3 ($\pm$4.8)% for patients with no ductus, 66.5 ($\pm$10.4)% for those with small PDA and 22.7 ($\pm$12.4)% for those with large ligated PDA.

Ventricular Septal Defect. Presence of small VSD had an effect on survival little better than absence of VSD, but this difference has a borderline statistical significance, while the presence of large VSD was significant in the negative sense. At 3 months of life survival was 82.5 ($\pm$3.9)% for patients with no VSD, 90.0 ($\pm$9.5)% for small VSD and 47.1 ($\pm$8.6)% for large VSD.

Left Ventricular Outflow Tract Obstruction. Presence of LVOTO had always a benefical effect: at 1 year survival was 54.2 ($\pm$5.3)% in patients with no obstruction, 84.4 ($\pm$8.3)% for trivial obstruction, 91.7 ($\pm$8.0)% for moderate obstruction and 90.9 ($\pm$8.7)% for severe obstruction.

Coarctation/Aortic Stenosis. Here the effects were diametrically opposite to those of LVOTO. Both patients with aortic stenosis died, and so all 6 patients with CoA non-corrected, and 4 of 6 patients who underwent surgery for CoA.

This epidemiological-statistical study, as already indicated, does not permit an absolute correlation between the several risk factors and survival; in other words we cannot assume that because a factor has a statistically significant effect on survival that alteration of that factor will alter survival in the manner predicted. But knowledge of the possible risk factors will permit, if possible, to modify them. Finally, to have tables of probability for survival at 6 months can help in knowing in advance which patients are at high risk, and consequently for which patients an earlier definitive surgery will be necessary.

In consideration of our results, the following conclusions can be drawn: (1) at-risk patients should have definitive repair within the first 6 months of life; (2) haemoglobin levels should be maintained, if necessary by transfusion; (3) persistent ductus arterious should be ligated, (4) earlier referral might improve overall survival.

Aldo Agnetti, MD, Clinica Pediatrica, Università degli Studi, I-43100 Parma (Italy)

Mod. Probl. Paediat., vol. 22, pp. 83–87 (Karger, Basel 1983)

Transposition of the Great Arteries

Mark R. de Leval

The Hospital for Sick Children, London, UK

First of all I would like to summarize our policy for transposition of the great arteries at Great Ormond Street. Between 1964 and 1978 the Mustard operation was the procedure of choice for patients with transposition of the great arteries in whom an intra-atrial repair was performed. In 1978, my colleague, Mr. *Stark*, started to perform Senning operations and I continued to do Mustard repairs until very recently. The intention was to try to compare two groups of patients operated upon using similar techniques and similar methods of myocardial protection. The results of this comparative study have not been completely analyzed, but our current thoughts are outlined in this paper.

This discussion will be limited to patients with simple transposition of the great arteries and intact ventricular septum. A balloon atrial septostomy is performed in the neonatal period. If they improve they are reinvestigated at the age of 4–5 months and an intra-atrial repair is done between 8–12 months of age. If the patients deteriorate they are restudied and an intra-atrial repair is carried out regardless of the age of the patient.

The technique of the Mustard procedure has changed over the years. Here we describe our current technique which consists of using a patch of pericardium trimmed into a trouser-like shape. Basically, we follow the suggestion made by Prof. *Brom* in trying to have a pericardial patch which will make up approximately two thirds of the circumference of the superior and the inferior venae cavae pathways. The operation is carried out on cardiopulmonary bypass, for most patients with direct cannulation of the superior and the inferior venae cavae. Cannulation is facilitated by a right-angled cannula. Two types of atrial incision may be performed, one a longitudinal incision in front of the crista terminalis performed in all children in whom we do not intend to enlarge the pulmonary venous atrium. For smaller infants and those patients under 6 months of age we perform an anteroposterior incision going down between the right upper and right lower pulmonary veins to enlarge the pulmonary venous atrium. Next, the remnant of the interatrial septum is excised. We routinely reendothelialize the raw area where the septum is excised and the trousershaped patch is inserted starting between the left pulmonary veins and the base of the left atrial appendage. The first suture line between the pulmonary veins and the left atrial appendage is carried laterally to the junction between the right upper pulmonary vein and the superior vena cava, the right lower pulmonary vein and the inferior vena cava. The second suture line starts at the remnant of the interatrial septum, again it is carried up above the SVC orifice and down above the IVC orifice keeping the coronary sinus in the pulmonary venous atrium.

In small infants, mainly under 3 months of age, the operation is performed with the aid of deep hypothermia and circulatory arrest with a single cannula in the right atrium. The atriotomy incision is an anteroposterior one which allows enlargement of the pulmonary venous atrium at the end of the procedure. We have used several materials to enlarge the pulmonary venous atrium: pericardium, xenograft pericardium, Dacron, and more recently Gore-Tex prosthesis.

I would like to discuss a few problems related to the early and long-term results of the Mustard procedure and compare them with the Senning procedure. The problems which have to be discussed are: (1) mortality (early and late), (2) preservation of the atrial function, (3) postoperative arrhythmias, and (4) late right ventricular function. The early mortality for the Mustard procedure has been 2% for the last few years. This is for the entire GOS (1964–1978). If we compare the mortality for the first series of Senning procedures done by Mr. *Stark*, we can see that up to May 1981 he had done 39 Sennings without any deaths from the TGA. There were 2 deaths among complex transpositions. If we look at atrial function after atrial repair: first of all I think that everyone will agree that after the Mustard operation or the Senning operation the venous pathways are only pathways but not reservoirs as a normal atrium is supposed to be. The atrium is made of two tubes which connect the cavae to the left ventricle. In order to assess the atrial function in patients who underwent the Senning and the Mustard operation, a member of our team, Dr. *Wyse*, studied in a group of patients operated in Leiden the jugular venous flow velocity using the Doppler technique. The comparative postoperative study included 24 patients; 16 underwent a Senning procedure and 8 a Mustard operation. All these patients were recatheterized in order to rule out any major hemodynamic anomaly. The left ventricular pressures were basically similar. The pulmonary artery pressure was within normal limits. There was a minimal gradient between the left ventricle and the pulmonary artery and there was no evidence of systemic venous obstruction. After Mustard, there is typically a forward flow to the right atrium only during the diastole with a loss of the forward flow during ventricular systole and of the reverse flow in atrial systole. In the Senning procedure the curve is nearly normal as there are two waves of forward flow, one corresponding to the ventricular systole, the second corresponding to the ventricular diastole and a reversed flow in the atrial systole. We believe that in the Senning procedure there is probably a preservation of the atrial function as a reservoir on one hand but also as a contractile chamber on the other. We have carried out three types of studies on arrhythmias after intra-atrial repair: the first two attempted to relate postoperative arrhythmias with the intraoperative procedure and the third study, which is not yet complete, consists of comparing 24-hour monitoring of patients carried out 2 weeks following a Senning or a Mustard procedure. The first study consisted of mapping the atria during the Mustard procedure. Intra-atrial mapping of the atrium before and after caval cannulation, atriotomy, excision of the atrial septum and placement of the atrial baffle was carried out in 32 patients. We had grids which represented the anatomic landmarks of the right atrium. After cannulation there are two preferential ways for the conduction to reach the atrioventricular node from the SA node. There is a preferential pathway along the crista terminalis which goes to the atrioventricular node. After a longitudinal incision, anterior to the crista terminalis, this pathway of faster conduction is preserved. For patients in whom the coronary sinus was included in the systemic venous atrium, there was an interruption of the fastest conduction along the posterior pathway in the area of the coronary sinus. The atrioventricular node remained activated by a zone of faster conduction along the roof of the tricuspid valve to reach the atrioventricular node. Following a transverse atriotomy incision there is complete interruption of this zone of faster conduction along the crista terminalis. Among the 32 patients studied, nodal rhythm was found in 4 on completion of the repair. They all had an interruption of the two pathways of faster conduction. These patients remained in junctional rhythm and arrhythmias but were basically in sinus rhythm most of the time. The second study consisted of following patients who had a 24-hour monitoring 2 weeks after the Mustard procedure. In that group there were 44 patients; 24 had simple transpositions and 20 complex transpositions of the great arteries. There were 6 sudden deaths among these 44 patients. The first patient was 10 months of age at the time of operation. The last ECG showed sinus rhythm and he also had sinus rhythm on the 24 hour monitoring. This patient had also undergone a ventricular septal defect closure. The second patient was in sinus rhythm on the 24-hour monitoring ECG. He had a Mustard plus closure of the VSD and a conduit inserted between the left ventricle and the pulmonary artery. The third patient died suddenly at the age of 17 years after palliative Mustard. These sudden deaths can of course be related to pulmonary vascular disease. There were 3 deaths among patients with simple transposition of the great arteries operated in infancy: 1 of them had remained in sinus rhythm throughout and 2 had arrhythmias during the perioperative period. The conclusion of this study is that it is very difficult to correlate arrhythmias with intraoperative procedures. However, it is also difficult to correlate late deaths with arrhythmias if we base our studies on 24-hour monitoring done in the early postoperative period. We now wonder if these arrhythmias could result from progressive fibrosis around the suture lines close of the conduction system. We have also compared patients who had a Senning procedure and patients with a Mustard procedure. So far, the incidence of arrhythmias on the 24-hour monitoring 2 weeks postoperatively is basically the same for the two procedures. The third type of complication which we have to consider is the incidence of venous obstruction. The incidence of pulmonary venous obstruction after Mustard has been very low and we believe that these obstructions are mainly related to technical problems. It is important to avoid placing the baffle too near the orifice of the right pulmonary veins. The suture line has to go back around the ostium of the superior and the inferior venae cavae to avoid ballooning of the patch above the right pulmonary veins. We have also reduced the incidence of pulmonary venous obstruction in small infants by enlarging the pulmonary venous atrium. We have been less successful in completely abolishing systemic venous obstructions. This incidence has been reduced by using the trouser-shaped baffle and also by using pericardium.

More recently I had 3 patients who did not show any evidence of caval obstruction following the Mustard procedure, but 3 years postoperatively, presented with venous obstruction. This has been my main reason for changing to the Senning procedure.

Finally one should consider the late functional results knowing that after intra-atrial repair the right ventricle has to serve the systemic circulation. It is well known that the morphology or at least the wall thickness of the right ventricle becomes the one of a left ventricle. We have not systematically restudied our patients after Mustard procedures. Dr. *Bonham-Carter* recently reviewed a group of 200 patients who underwent Mustard procedure between 1965 and 1971. In that group of patients there were 35 hospital deaths, 15 were lost to follow-up. Among the 150 patients who survived there were 30 late deaths, i.e. 20% of the patients. The analysis of these late deaths is as follows: 17 were unknown, 5 were sudden and probably related to late arrhythmias, 6 were related to patch contraction and 6 patients died for reasons unrelated to the cardiac anomaly. We have also studied the exercise tolerance in a group of 20 patients after the Mustard procedure. The study has shown that the exercise tolerance is reduced in patients who had Mustard procedure compared to normal children, but this does not say that it is because the left ventricle is serving the systemic circulation.

Finally we have also reviewed, although only with a questionnaire, a group of patients who were operated upon in earlier years. They were reviewed 5–10 years postoperatively and in that group there were only 44% with excellent results. These patients had a normal exercise tolerance, at least according to the questionnaire and have a normal heart size on chest X-ray, are in sinus rhythm and do not take any medication. In conclusion, therefore, the results of the Mustard procedure are satisfactory but the right ventricular function must also be assessed if we want to look at the long-term results. Late arrhythmias remain a problem not only for the Mustard but also for the Senning operation.

M.R. de Leval, MD, The Hospital for Sick Children, Great Ormond Street, London WC1N 3JH (UK)

Mod. Probl. Paediat., vol. 22, pp. 88–91 (Karger, Basel 1983)

Mustard's Operation for 'Simple' Transposition of the Great Arteries (TGA)

Gian Piero Piccoli

Royal Liverpool Children's Hospital, Liverpool, England

At the Royal Liverpool Children's Hospital, between January 1970 and January 1980, 80 consecutive patients, ranging in age from 42 days to 13 years (mean = 15 months) underwent Mustard's operation for 'simple' transposition of the great arteries. There were 2 early deaths, one of which was due to cerebral damage, while the other was caused by inferior vena cava thrombosis. The early postoperative period was completely uneventful in 56 patients, while the remainder had one or more major complications (table I). Standard electrocardiograms revealed 2 main types of dysrhythmias in 29 cases (table II). 18 patients suffered transient atrioventricular (AV) conduction dysfunction, while in another 6 infants this type of arrhythmia persisted at discharge. 5 cases showed sinus node-atrial dysfunction, which was temporary in 2 and permanent in the other 3.

At follow-up (mean = 4.5 years) 74 % of survivors were symptom-free. Late dysrhythmias were recorded in 11 patients. AV conduction disturbances were present in 6 cases, while sinus node-atrial dysfunction occurred in 5 (table II). These arrhythmias did not prevent the children from leading a normal life. Re-investigation was performed in 13 symptomatic cases. These haemodynamic data, combined with the clinical examination in the others, were used to assess several types of late complications, although these were not always associated with clinical deterioration (table III). Pulmonary venous obstruction was encountered in 6 cases, 4 of whom underwent successful plastic enlargement of the pulmonary atrium; the fifth patient died at re-operation, while the sixth died at home. Superior vena cava obstruction occurred in 7 cases. In 3 patients this was associated with a mild degree of tricuspid valve incompetence, and in 3 others with a residual shunt at atrial level. 2 of these patients underwent successful surgical revision of their inter-

Table I. Early complications (22 patients affected)

Complications	Incidence
Low cardiac output	6
Respiratory failure	5
Chest infection	8
Cerebral damage	4[1]
Surgical bleeding	3
Wound infection	4
Unilateral phrenic nerve paralysis	7[2]
Renal failure	1

[1] In 2 patients cerebral lesions were present pre-operatively.
[2] Phrenic unilateral nerve paralysis was temporary in 5 cases and permanent in 2.

Table II. Early and late postoperative dysrhythmias

	Temporary early dysrhythmias	Permanent early dysrhythmias	Late dysrhythmias
Sinus node-atrial dysfunction	2	3[1]	5[1]
Atrioventricular conduction dysfunction	18	6[2, 3]	6[2, 4]
Intraventricular conduction dysfunction		9	15
Total	20	18	26

[1] 1 patient had sick syndrome pre-operatively.
[2] 2 patients had first degree atrioventricular block pre-operatively.
[3] 2 cases with complete atrioventricular block.
[4] 3 cases with complete atrioventricular block.

atrial baffle. Small residual ventricular septal defects were present in 4 cases, being associated in 1 with tricuspid valve incompetence and in another with residual shunt at atrial level. None of these children had symptoms warranting operation. Isolated tricuspid valve incompetence was demonstrated by the right ventricular angiography only in 1 case. The systemic ventricular

Table III. Late complications

	Number of patients	Re-operation
PVs obstruction	6	5
Moderate SVC obstruction, Mild TVI	3	
Residual interatrial shunt, SVC obstruction	3	2
Isolated SVC obstruction	1	
Residual small VSD	2	
Residual small VSD, mild TVI	1	
Residual interatrial shunt, interventricular shunt, mild LVOTO	1	
Mild LVOTO	3	
Isolated TVI	1	
Cerebral damage	4[1]	
Total	25	7

PV = Pulmonary veins; SVC = superior vena cava; TVI = tricuspid valve incompetence; VSD = ventricular septal defect; LVOTO = left ventricular outflow tract obstruction.
[1] In 2 patients cerebral damage was present pre-operatively.

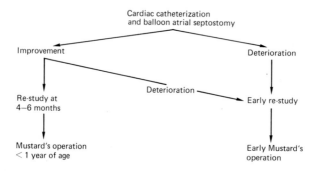

Fig. 1. Surgical management for patients with simple transposition of the great arteries.

function was assessed in those patients who were re-investigated. The degree of right ventricular impairment was always related to the severity of the associated complications, existing in 1 case only as primary feature. Only 1 infant, 7 months old, presented clinical features of primitive right ventrucular failure and he died at home, 4 months after the operation. In our unit, the policy which is adopted for cases with 'simple' transposition of the great arteries is illustrated in figure 1.

In conclusion, our early mortality rate (2.5%) and our late results (3 late deaths, 6% overall mortality rate and three quarters of survivors leading normal lives) compare favourably with the results achieved in other centres performing different types of physiological or anatomical corrections. Therefore, at the present time, there seems to be no good reason to alter our surgical policy in this group of patients.

Gian Piero Piccoli, MD, Ospedale Specializzato Regionale, "G.M.Lancisi", Via Baccarani 6, I–60100 Ancona (Italy)

Mod. Probl. Paediat., vol. 22, pp. 92–96 (Karger, Basel 1983)

Transposition of the Great Arteries: Clinical and Instrumental Evaluation after Senning Correction

Antonio Castellani

Department of Cardiology, Ospedale Civile di Vicenza, Vicenza, Italy

Complete transposition of the great arteries (TGA) is one of the congenital cardiac defects whose prognosis is more changed because of the striking innovation in treatment in these last years. From January 1977 to August 1981, TGA was found in 8.7 % of haemodynamic studies for paediatric age performed in our laboratory. We examined 56 TGA (table I), 32 of which (1st group) had intact interventricular septum and 24 (2nd group) were associated with a defect of the interventricular septum (VSD). In the first group 24 TGA were isolated, 4 associated to a patent ductus arteriosus (PDA), 2 to pulmonary artery stenosis. In the second group 11 TGA were associated to the only VSD; various anomalies were present in the remaining cases. In most of the cases, during the catheterization, an atrial septostomy according to Rashkind was performed; palliative surgery in 11 cases – because of the persistence of serious cyanosis or because of its reappearing some time after septostomy – was carried out, with 9 % mortality.

The definitive 'physiological' correction was performed on 31 patients (table II); 30 Senning procedures and one Mustard procedure were carried out. 25 simple TGA and 6 TGA $\pm$ VSD were corrected (in 4 cases the VSD was closed through atria, in 2 cases by ventriculotomy). The body weight varied from 3.06 to 11.4 kg (mean 6.43); the age varied from 2 days to 23 months (mean 8.6 months).

Surgical mortality (2/31) was 6.45 %; in a first case it was due to low output syndrome, in a second case to renal insufficiency secondary to CEC. There was no late mortality. Among the 29 survivors, 26 have been periodically clinically and instrumentally evaluated; the last 3, recently operated, have not yet entered the follow-up. In 15 cases the haemodynamic study was repeated with right cardiac catheterization. The follow-up varied from

Table I. Transposition of the great arteries (56 patients; incidence 8.7%)

32 transposition of the great arteries without ventricular septal defect	25 transposition of the great arteries
	4 transposition of the great arteries + patent ductus arteriosus
	2 transposition of the great arteries + pulmonary stenosis
24 transposition of the great arteries with ventricular septal defect	11 transposition of the great arteries + ventricular septal defect
	5 transposition of the great arteries + ventricular septal defect + pulmonary stenosis
	3 transposition of the great arteries + ventricular septal defect + pulmonary hypertension
	1 transposition of the great arteries + ventricular septal defect + tricuspid atresia
	1 transposition of the great arteries + ventricular septal defect + pulmonary atresia
	1 transposition of the great arteries + ventricular septal defect + right ventricle and aortic root hypoplasia
	2 transposition of the great arteries + ventricular septal defect + D.O.R.V.

Table II. Transposition of the great arteries

Palliative surgery	(11 patients)	mortality	9%	
Corrective surgery	(31 patients)	mortality	6.45%	(2/31)
		late mortality	–	–

Senning procedure	30
Mustard	1
Survivors	29
Clinical follow-up	26
Haemodynamic checking	15

Table III. Transposition of the great arteries: arrhythmias after Senning correction (26)

	0–24 h	Discharge	Follow-up (3–24 months)
Atrial premature beats	12	3	1
Ventricular premature beats	–	–	–
Atrial rhythm (not sinus)	1	–	–
Junctional rhythm	4	–	–
Arterioventricular block 1, 2	2	–	–
Arterioventricular block 3	–	–	–
RBB block	2	–	–
LBB block	–	–	–

Table IV. Transposition of the great arteries: Postoperative catheterization after Senning correction

No.	Months after correction	SVC mean	IVC mean	NRA mean	LV syst.	LV end diast.	PA syst.	PA mean	PW mean	LV–PA gradient
1	42	8	8	8	88	12	20	15	–	68
2	9	7	6	5	32	7	28	15	–	4
3	20	9	10	9	66	8	64	26	15	2
4	25	6	5	5	30	5	24	19	–	6
5	13	7	7	5	30	5	–	–	–	–
6	1	5	5	5	28	8	24	11	–	4
7	40	3	4	4	27	5	22	12	–	5
8	6	5	5	5	22	5	18	8	–	4
9	21	4	3	3	38	5	35	15	10	3
10	8	8	7	8	32	8	30	12	8	2
11	13	6	7	6	23	7	22	10	–	1
12	9	6	6	6	23	5	20	8	–	3
13	22	8	6	7	30	7	30	22	13	–
14	10	4	4	4	25	5	24	15	–	1
15	8	3	4	3	22	5	–	–	–	–

3 to 42 months after the operation. Clinically all the patients were in good condition, they did not show cyanosis and no diastolic or continuous murmurs were heard. From the radiological point of view, only 2 patients showed moderate pulmonary congestion. All the children, after correction, were under digitalis and/or diuretic treatment for about 2 months; 2 among

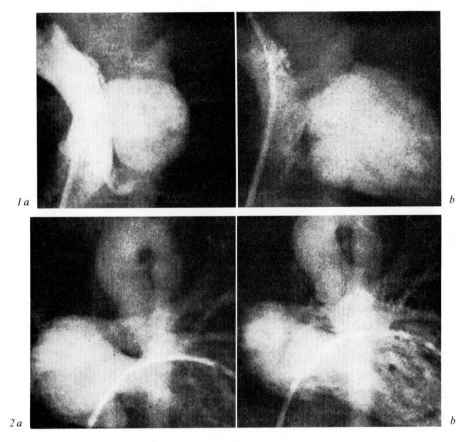

Fig. 1. The new right atrium: *a* atrial diastole; *b* atrial systole.
Fig. 2. The new left atrium: *a* atrial diastole; *b* atrial systole.

them are still in care for a moderate heart failure. The check-up of rhythm and conduction disorder was carried out by regular electrocardiograms; it was impossible for us to carry out a continuous electrocardiogram for 24 h; this began only recently.

Table III shows the incidence of the arrhythmias and conduction delays during the first 24 h after the operation, at discharge, and at the following check-up. All the patients were discharged with sinus rhythm, and in 3 cases with atrial premature beats still present; these beats were only present in 1 case at the following check-up (after 3 months).

The application of a pacemaker was never necessary. 1 patient, who had an asystolia when the anaesthesia was induced and reanimated, later showed an electrocardiographic pattern of inferior and lateral necrosis which has not presented, for the time being, peculiar consequences.

The haemodynamic check-up was always carried out by a balloon catheter in order to reach easily the pulmonary artery and not to run the risk of damaging the new atrial structures (table IV). The usual taking of blood samples never gave evidence of shunts. No pressure gradients resulted between venae cavae and the venous atrium. The gradient between the left ventricle and pulmonary artery was significant in only 1 case and was not present at pre-operative study. We checked the wedge pulmonary capillary pressure when the pulmonary artery pressure exceeded 30 mm Hg.

Angiographies have been carried out in the pulmonary artery or in the left ventricle and in the superior vena cava in order to check possible vascular stenosis or obstructions and the contractility (fig. 1–2) of the new atria and of the ventricles. A left heart catheterization has never been carried out.

Conclusions

The Senning procedure mortality is, at worst, like the Mustard procedure; to its advantage venous obstructions and rhythm or conduction disorders are rare. We can presume, for the Senning procedure, a better future, on the basis of a possible better development and contractility of the new atria, constituted mostly of tissues which are already present in the normal atria and which maintain, therefore, a proper muscular tone; internodal connections seem to be, moreover, better respected.

The doubt of the future endurance of the tricuspid valve and of the right ventricle are common to Mustard's and Senning's procedures; only a long-term follow-up will clear it. Our limited casuistry, our incomplete data and our limited follow-up enable us to make, at the present, only these remarks, however rather encouraging.

Antonio Castellani, MD, Divisione di Cardiologia, Ospedale Civile di Vicenza, I-36100 Vicenza (Italy)

Mod. Probl. Paediat., vol. 22, pp. 97–109 (Karger, Basel 1983)

Surgical Repair of Total Anomalous Pulmonary Venous Return: Early and Late Results

Peter B. Mansfield, Dale G. Hall, Edward A. Rittenhouse, Stanley J. Stamm, S. Paul Herndon

Children's Orthopedic Hospital and Medical Center, Seattle, Wash., USA

Introduction

Untreated total anomalous pulmonary venous return (TAPVR) leads to death in the majority of cases before the first year of age [1, 2]. The surgical success of repair of this complex defect has slowly been improving over the last two decades. Mortality rates as high as 60–70% between 1960 and 1970 were reduced to the 10–40% range by the mid 1970s [3–8]. Specific centers by 1980 were reporting 12–14% hospital mortality [6, 9, 10].

As techniques have improved, including preoperative diagnosis, operative repair and postoperative care, patients with significant elevation of pulmonary vascular resistance have begun to survive for long-term follow-up. Late deaths have become a significant part of the risk in this congenital heart defect [7, 8]. All patients with TAPVR seen at Children's Orthopedic Hospital and Medical Center from 1972 to 1981 comprise the patients in this study of early and late results of surgical repair.

Clinical Material

23 patients with total anomalous pulmonary venous return have been treated in this 9-year interval. The distribution of anatomic types of TAPVR is shown in table I [11]. There were 13 males and 10 females. All were symptomatic. Presenting symptoms included varying degrees of tachypnea, congestive failure, cyanosis and hepatomegaly. All had right ventricular hypertrophy for age on EKG. Patients with increased pulmonary flow had large hearts and prominent pulmonary vascular congestion. Patients with decreased pulmonary flow or marked lymphatic obstruction had normal or small hearts and usually a typical reticular pattern on chest X-ray [12]. These were almost always

Table I. Anatomic sites of total anomalous pulmonary venous return

	Patients	Totals	(%)
Supracardiac		6	(26)
SVC	1		
Left vertical vein	5		
Cardiac		7	(30)
coronary sinus	5		
RA	2		
Infracardiac	10	10	(44)
Mixed	0	0	
		23	

infracardiac type defects and frequently presented in the poorest clinical condition. These severely obstructed patients presented more frequently shortly after birth than the patients with high pulmonary flow and insignificant pulmonary venous obstruction. Echocardiography has been helpful in the differential diagnosis in many of these cases [13].

Late referral of patients with TAPVR is common because of lack of murmurs, confusing chest X-rays, and modest other distinguishing features. This gives time for failure to thrive to become apparent. Those patients that presented at less than 1 month of age, regardless of anatomic type, fell between the 10th and 90th percentile for both height and weight with the exception of a single premature infant. Those who presented at 2 months all were less than the 10th percentile by weight. Those presenting at 3 months or later were all well below the 5th percentile both in height and weight. Subsequent follow-up has shown that those patients whose pulmonary vascular resistence remains continuously elevated postoperatively continue to have severe problems of failure to thrive.

Our current approach to TAPVR is immediate cardiac catheterization upon suggestion of the diagnosis. If infracardiac (type III) anomalous return is found, a balloon atrial septostomy is performed and surgery is undertaken as soon as possible, usually within 24 h. If the venous return is supracardiac (type I) or cardiac (type II) and the atrial septum is not restrictive, we usually wait until 3–6 months of age to perform a total open repair. If congestive symptoms are not manageable medically, surgery is undertaken at any time. If in type I and type II the atrial septum is restrictive, a balloon atrial septostomy is performed and, if pulmonary venous return is still obstructive, immediate surgery is undertaken. If the balloon septostomy relieves the obstruction, elective surgery at 3–6 months of age is planned. Table II defines the ages at catheterization and surgery, and the indications for the timing of the operation.

Surgical Technique

With the exception of the balloon atrial septostomy in specific cases, total anomalous pulmonary venous return is not a congenital defect which is amenable to palliative surgery. Early in our series we used cardiopulmonary bypass without circulatory arrest at approximately 24 °C to repair these defects. We now prefer hypothermic, circulatory

Table II. Age at initial catheterization and operative indications – TAPVR

Type	Obstructed	Age cath.	op.	Operative indications
Supracardiac	yes	1 d	1 d	obstr.
		1 d	1 d	obstr.
		18 d	18 d	obstr.
	no	1 d	3 mo	routine
		3 mo	1 yr	routine
		12 yr	12 yr	routine
Cardiac	yes	8 d	8 d	obstr.
	no	11 d	awaiting	routine
		35 d	36 d	↑ ↑ pulm. flow
		85 d	89 d	↑ ↑ pulm. flow
		89 d	103 d	routine
		96 d	114 d	assoc. lesions: VSD
		167 d	170 d	routine-remote refer
Infracardiac	yes	1 d	1 d	obstr. $R_p:R_s$ 1.4
		1 d	1 d	obstr.
		6 d	6 d	obstr. $R_p:R_s$ 0.45
		8 d	9 d	obstr.
		10 d	11 d	obstr. moribund
		16 d	18 d	obstr.
		21 d	22 d	obstr.
		48 d	48 d	S/P arrest, moribund
		49 d	50 d	obstr. $R_p:R_s$ 0.5
		85 d	86 d	obstr. moribund S/P arrest ×2

Table III. Influence of TAPVR type and PDA on pulmonary artery peak pressure

Type	PDA	Patients	Average peak PAP ($\pm$ 1SD)[1]	Average peak PAP ($\pm$ 1SD)[1]
Supracardiac	yes	2	65	68 (18)
	no	4	70 (22)	
Cardiac	yes	1	60	52 (6.4)
	no	6	51 (6)	
Infracardiac	yes	3	69 (12)	79 (17)
	no	7	83 (17)	

[1] Standard deviation (70% confidence limits).

arrest using low room temperatures for initial cooling and brief cardiopulmonary bypass to bring the patient to approximately 18 °C at which time circulatory arrest is instituted. Arrest time is usually short. Rewarming to a rectal temperature of approximately 31 °C is accomplished before coming off bypass.

When a ductus is present it is closed only after bypass has commenced because it prevents the pulmonary arterial hypertension from exceeding systemic levels. 6 of our patients had a patent ductus and the average peak pulmonary artery pressure was lower in these cases than in those 17 patients without a patent ductus (table III). Location and size of the pulmonary venous return also determines the peak pulmonary artery pressure which may be present. Cardiac (type II) lesions usually have the least pulmonary venous obstruction and therefore the lowest average peak pulmonary artery pressure.

We repair cardiac (type II) return to the coronary sinus using the technique suggested by *Van Praagh* et al. [14]. We repair right atrial venous return using pericardial baffles to deflect the blood to the left atrium, usually through an enlarged atrial septal defect or excised patent foramen ovale. There were no mixed venous return (type IV) cases in this series. The surgical repair of supracardiac or infracardiac defects is similar because there is usually a confluence of the pulmonary veins behind the pericardium which can be anastomosed directly to the left atrium and the anomalous communication to the systemic venous return closed.

The literature is replete with descriptions of the varying sizes of the left atrium and the left ventricle in cases of TAPVR [15–17]. We have found it clinically difficult to determine which patients can tolerate closure of their atrial septum or require enlargement of their left atrium in order to survive. Since balloon atrial septostomy used in transposition of the great vessels usually has relatively insignificant flow by 2–5 years of age, we now routinely do balloon atrial septostomy for patients of type I supracardiac or type III infracardiac TAPVR regardless of whether there is obvious obstruction or not [18–22]. The repair for both these defects is similar and is shown in figures 1–3.

Following an initial balloon atrial septostomy the patient is ready for surgery. Because episodes of increased pulmonary vascular resistance occur in association with acidosis, base deficits, hypercarbia and hypoxia, we do our utmost to avoid these situations by anticipating their occurrence. The operating room is cooled so the patient's temperature will drop during preoperative preparations. Immediate sternotomy followed by single

---

Fig. 1. The configuration of infracardiac (type III) TAPVR is shown entering the portal system with stenosis at the entry point. These patients have initial balloon atrial septostomy performed at catheterization and are immediately referred for surgery.

Fig. 2. Preparation for the repair of infracardiac TAPVR includes room cooling followed by core cooling to 18 °C and total circulatory arrest. A small vent placed in the left ventricle decompresses the left heart and left atrium and when manipulated nicely defines the limits of the left atrium for the anastomosis. On the right the heart has been rotated superiorly, the confluent pulmonary veins exposed behind the pericardium and great care is taken to select the appropriate incision both in the small left atrium and the confluent veins. Almost always an anastomosis of at least 1 cm in length done with interrupted technique can be performed.

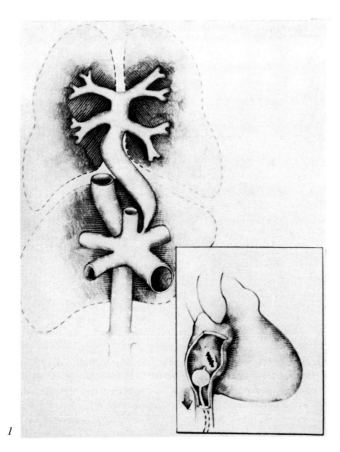

1

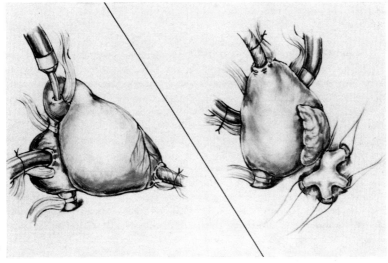

2

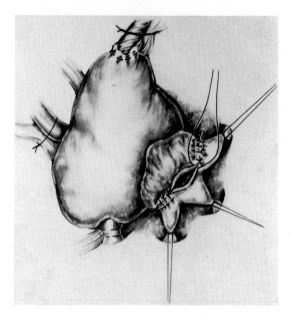

Fig. 3. The anastomosis between the confluent pulmonary veins and the left atrium is almost complete. The heart will be filled with iced saline to help remove air via the left ventricular vent. Cardiopulmonary bypass is reinitiated, the patient warmed to a rectal temperature of 31 °C and removed from bypass. The atrial septum is left open. We have not had to surgically close any atrial defect created by a balloon septostomy in these patients.

atrial cannulation and core cooling to 18 °C precede total circulatory arrest. A small left ventricular vent is slipped up through the mitral valve into the left atrium. We usually dissect out the common pulmonary veins during core cooling. The apex of the heart is rotated superiorly (fig. 2) and we very carefully select the line of incision on the left atrium and the confluent pulmonary vein so that when the heart is rotated back into its normal position there will be no tension or torsion at the anastomotic site. We have found it always possible to create an anastomosis of more than 1 cm in length frequently extending out along one of the major pulmonary veins toward the left lung. With the ductus controlled if patent, and each pulmonary vein individually secured, the incisions and *interrupted* anastomosis using 6–0 or 7–0 sutures are performed. Upon completion iced saline is injected into the pulmonary venous system to help clear air from the left atrium out the left ventricular vent which is then pulled to the left ventricular apex. Cardiopulmonary bypass and rewarming is initiated to a rectal temperature of 31 °C. Temporary atrial and ventricular pacing wires are left in place and the atrial septum is left open as a relief valve for the left heart. The CVP line is thus a monitor of left atrial pressure.

Postoperative Care

With the exception of a single case with an associated severe hypoplastic left heart and hypolastic aortic arch, we have been able to maintain adequate cardiac output following repair in all these cases. Several techniques have helped in the postoperative period to increase cardiac output. All measures previously mentioned to avoid precipitating sudden increased pulmonary vascular resistance are employed [10, 23]. Rapid atrial pacing to increase cardiac output when stroke volume or left atrial volume may be limiting has been of assistance with several patients. We use Levophed and Regitine in a combination which slightly increases peripheral vascular resistance rather than unloading what may be a volume or stroke volume limited left heart during the first 12–36 h [10]. We have found the left heart to enlarge rapidly by serial echo examinations and continued special support is rarely needed after 2 or 3 days.

Results

Table IV shows the mortality versus the type of TAPVR. The details of each patient who did not survive are documented in table V. There were 6 patients with supracardiac (type I) return with no operative deaths and 1 hospital death which occurred 2 months following surgery. There were no late deaths in this group. There were also 6 patients with cardiac return (type II). There were no operative or hospital deaths in this group. There was 1 late death at approximately 10 months of age from continued elevated pulmonary vascular resistance.

There were 10 patients with infracardiac (type III) defects with 1 operative death (hypoplastic left heart), 1 hospital death 12 days after surgery from CNS damage sustained during two cardiac arrests and a 1-hour resuscitation prior to Children's Orthopedic Hospital and Medical Center admission, and there was 1 late death at 4 years from a progressive increase in pulmonary vascular resistance (cor pulmonale).

The hospital mortality was 3 patients in 22 cases or 14% and an additional 11% mortality as late deaths from among the remaining patients. Symptoms from persistant elevation in pulmonary vascular resistance were always present within 3–5 months from the time of surgical repair. In evaluating this problem the use of the ratio of the pulmonary vascular resistance to systemic resistance has no application in patients who are operated on under a week or two of age. This is because the ratio appears to diminish because the mean arterial systemic pressures increase with age. A better way of following pulmonary vascular resistance is to determine the absolute value of pulmonary vascular resistance and compare it to the patient's own previous values.

Table IV. Mortality versus type of TAPVR

Type	Patients	Operative death	Hospital death	Late death
Supracardiac	6	0	1	0
Cardiac[1]	6	0	0	1
Infracardiac	10	1	1	1
	22	1	2	2

[1] 1 patient awaits repair.

Influences on Mortality and Morbidity

We found no significant influence of age at operation on subsequent mortality. The two most important factors contributing to ultimate death, whether it be hospital or late, were the presence of preoperative and post-operative elevation of pulmonary vascular resistance. A patent ductus arteriosus which kept pulmonary artery pressures low preoperatively did not protect one of the patients who died at 4 years of age from elevated pulmonary vascular resistance and cor pulmonale. Although the anatomy of the pulmonary arterial obstruction which causes the elevated pulmonary vascular resistance is well described [24] why it occurs in 1 patient and not another is not clear. It may be of note that the 2 late deaths and the patient who died in the hospital 2 months after surgery due to an elevated pulmonary vascular resistance all had severe pulmonary lymphatic obstruction with exceedingly stiff lungs and markedly widened pulmonary septa which made the surface of the lungs look like deeply ridged pigskin. If the surgical repair does not relieve this lymphatic obstruction it may lead to interstitial scarring and pulmonary vascular obstruction. Chronic lymphatic stasis causes scarring in other areas of the body such as the extremities.

All the patients with prolonged elevated pulmonary resistance were re-catheterized. All anastomoses were crossed with end hole catheters and no gradients were found. There were no pulmonary venous strictures. Pulmonary wedge pressures were normal in every case suggesting pulmonary arteriolar obstruction as the etiology of the pulmonary vascular resistance elevation. We have had no cases of anastomonic obstruction in this series. Associated cardiac lesions incompatible with survival and severe CNS damage before repair are understandable causes of mortality.

Table V. Cause of mortality – TAPVR

Type	Timing	Preop. status	Age at op.	at death	Cause of death
Supracardiac	HD	clinically critical PAP 78/45 $R_p:R_s$ 1.4	< 1 d	64 d	chronic pulmonary interstitial pneumonitis no △ in initial ↑ ↑ PVR pulmonary lymphatic obstr.
Cardiac	LD	clinically stable ↑ heart size, ↑ liver ↑ ↑ pulm.flow, PAP 60/40	8 d	306 d	continued ↑ PVR cor pulmonale no venous or anastomotic obstruction at 2nd cath. (wedge normal)
Infracardiac	OD	intubated, paralyzed, severe CHF before transfer, HLH syndrome by echo	11 d	11 d	associated lesion: hypoplastic left heart aortic arch hypoplasia
	HD	cardiac arrests ×2 1-hour resuscitation, seizures, intubated, moribund before transfer	48 d	60 d	preop. CNS damage CV status postop. OK
	LD	clinically stable reticular X-ray EKG: RVH PAP 55/30 PDA (large)	< 1 d	4 yr	progressive ↑ PVR cor pulmonale no venous or anastomotic obstruction at 2nd cath. (wedge normal)

HD = Hospital death; LD = late death; OD = operative death; PAP = pulmonary artery pressure; PVR = pulmonary vascular resistance; CHF = Congestive Heart Failure; HLH = hypoplastic left heart; CV = cardiovascular; RVH = right ventricular hypoplasia; PDA = patent ductus arteriosus.

Table VI. Follow-up of hospital survivors – TAPVR

Type	Hospital survival, %	Late death	Alive and well	↑ PVR (stable)	Follow-up	
					mean, years	range
Supracardiac (6)	83	–	5	0	3	(9 mo to 8 years)
Cardiac (6)	100	1	5	0	2.8	(1.5–5 years)
Infracardiac (10)	80	1	6	1	4.9	(0.1–9 years)

Long-Term Follow-Up

Table VI shows the long-term follow-up of the 19 hospital survivors. There were no late deaths in the supracardiac group and all 5 are alive and well without evidence of increased pulmonary vascular resistance over a mean follow-up of 3 years. There was 1 late death in the cardiac group, a result of continued elevated pulmonary vascular resistance. The remaining 5 are alive and well with a mean follow-up time of 2.8 years. There was 1 late death in the infracardiac group 4 years following surgery also due to an elevated pulmonary vascular resistance. 1 patient has a moderate increase in pulmonary vascular resistance which has been stable for the last several years. That patient remains in the 75% in height and weight and is fully active. 6 others are alive and well. Mean follow-up for the infracardiac group is 4.9 years.

Discussion

As this and other papers have demonstrated [25, 26] the operative and hospital mortality for the surgical repair of TAPVR has diminished in recent years. When one reviews the remaining major contributing factors to mortality, we are really left with: (1) late referral creating a sicker child at operative correction, (2) associated cardiac lesions (usually a ventricular septal defect, VSD) which may be incompatible with life (hypoplastic left heart), (3) persistent elevation of pulmonary vascular resistance postoperatively, and (4) pulmonary venous obstruction reported [25] but not seen in this series.

Late referrals occur because a TAPVR is actually very rarely seen and it is unusual for a pediatrician to see more than one in his life-time. In addition, the chest X-ray picture is quite consistent with idiopathic respiratory distress syndrome or chronic viral pneumonitis. Murmurs when present are usually soft and not alarming and heart size is frequently normal or slightly small.

Cyanosis of a significant nature is usually a late finding. Education must be the answer here. Because of our referral pattern we have had 2 patients sent to us on the first day or two of life because the referring physician had seen a previous case. The characteristic reticular pattern of the infracardiac type with an associated small heart is a clue that should not be missed.

The most common associated lesions are patent ductus arteriosus which if large keeps the peak pulmonary artery pressure down to systemic levels and an occassional ventricular septal defect which should be fixed at the time of the total repair. Our case of hypoplastic left heart and aortic arch is distinctly unusual.

The biggest problem is the persistance of pulmonary hypertension and pulmonary vascular resistance. One must not be fooled by a dropping $R_p:R_s$ ratio when in fact the R_p is not changing with time. The 2 late deaths due to elevated pulmonary vascular resistance did not alter the resistance with oxygen. The 1 patient with elevated pulmonary vascular resistance who remains alive and is doing well does respond dramatically to oxygen with lowering of his pulmonary vascular resistance. We have found in other patients with elevated pulmonary vascular resistance that blood pH can play a significant role in controlling pulmonary vascular resistance fluctuations. We try to keep the pH at 7.5 or 7.6 in critical cases [23].

In all of our postoperative catheterizations of patients with elevated pulmonary artery resistances the obstruction appears to be on the pulmonary arteriolar side. There have been no anastomotic or pulmonary venous obstructions or pressure gradients and the wedge pressures are normal in all these patients [24]. How to permanently reverse these arteriolar changes would be a major step forward in congenital heart surgery.

Pulmonary venous obstruction both at the anastomosis and above it in the pulmonary veins has been described [25]. It is also a dangerous postoperative condition which can lead to sudden death. Since most of these anastomoses are made in small infants we believe interrupted suture technique is most appropriate to avoid the possibility of anastomotic strictures that continuous suture techniques can create.

Patients who avoid the above pitfalls seem to do quite well. Problems from elevated pulmonary vascular resistance are usually apparent within the first year following surgery and we have not seen such problems appear after that time.

References

1 Gomes, M.M.R.; Feldt, R.H.; McGoon, D.C.; Danielson, G.K.: Total anomalous pulmonary venous connection. J.thorac.cardiovasc.Surg. *60:* 116 (1970).

2 Applebaum, A.; Kirklin, J.W.; Pacifico, A.D.; Bargeron, L.M.: The surgical treatment of total anomalous pulmonary venous connection. Israel J.med.Scis *11:* 89 (1975).

3 Wukasch, D.C.; Deutsch, M.; Reul, G.J.; Hallman, G.L.; Cooley, D.A.: Total anomalous pulmonary venous return. Ann.thorac.Surg. *19:* 622 (1975).

4 Gersony, W.M.; Bowman, F.O.; Steeg, C.N.; Hayes, C.J.; Jesse, M.J.; Malm, J.R.: Management of total anomalous pulmonary venous drainage in early infancy. Circulation *43, 44* (Suppl.1): 119–124 (1971).

5 Hayes, C.J.; Gersony, W.M.; Griffiths, S.P.; Steeg, C.N.; Bowman, F.O., Jr.; Malm, J.R.: Results of correction of total anomalous pulmonary venous connections in infancy. Adv.Cardiol. *11:* 36–42 (1974).

6 Higashino, S.M.; Shaw, G.G.; May, I.A.; Ecker, R.R.: Total anomalous pulmonary venous drainage below the diaphragm. J.thorac.cardiovasc.Surg. *68:* 711–718 (1974).

7 Katz, N.M.; Kirklin, J.W.; Pacifico, A.D.: Concepts and practices in surgery for total anomalous pulmonary venous connection. Ann.thoracic.Surg. *25:* 479 (1978).

8 Whight, C.M.; Barratt-Boyes, B.G.; Calder, A.L.; Neutze, J.M.; Brandt, P.W.T.: Total anomalous pulmonary venous connection. J.thorac.cardiovasc.Surg. *75:* 52 (1978).

9 Turley, K.; Tucker, W.Y.; Ullyot, D.J.; Ebert, P.A.: Total anomalous pulmonary venous connection in infancy: influence of age and type of lesion. Am.J.cardiol. *45:* 92 (1980).

10 Mansfield, P.B.; Hall, D.G.; Rittenhouse, E.A.; Sauvage, L.R.; Stamm, S.S.; Herndon, S.P.; Furman, E.C.: Cardiac surgery under age two years. J.thorac.cardiovasc.Surg. *77:* 816–825 (1979).

11 Darling, R.C.; Rothney, W.B.; Craig, J.M.: Total pulmonary venous drainage into the right side of the heart. Lab.Invest. *6:* 44 (1957).

12 Robinson, A.E.; Chen, J.T.T.; Bradford, W.D.; Lester, R.G.: Kerley B lines in total anomalous pulmonary venous connection below the diaphragm (type III). Am. J.Cardiol. *24:* 436 (1969).

13 Paquet, M.; Gutgesell, H.: Echocardiographic features of total anomalous pulmonary venous connection. Circulation *51:* 599 (1975).

14 Van Praagh, R.; Harken, A.H.; Delisle, G.; Ando, M.; Gross, R.E.: Total anomalous pulmonary venous drainage to the coronary sinus. J.thorac.cardiovasc.Surg. *64:* 132–135 (1972).

15 Graham, T.P., Jr.; Jarmakani, J.M.; Canent, R.V.: Left heart volume characteristics with a right ventricular volume overload. Circulation *65:* 389 (1972).

16 Coussement, A.M.; Gooding, C.A.; Carlsson, E.: Left atrial volume, shape, and movement in total anomalous pulmonary venous return. Radiology *107:* 139 (1973).

17 Bove, K.E.; Geiser, E.A.; Meyer, R.A.: The left ventricle in anomalous pulmonary venous return. Archs Path. *99:* 522 (1975).

18 Miller, W.W.; Rashkind, W.J.: Palliative treatment of total anomalous pulmonary venous drainage by balloon atrial septostomy. Lancet *Aug.17:* 387 (1968).

19 Serratto, M.; Bucheleres, H.G.; Bicoff, P.; Miller, R.A.; Hastreiter, A.R.: Palliative balloon atrial septostomy for total anomalous pulmonary venous connection in infancy. J.Pediat. *73*: 734 (1968).

20 Silove, E.D.; Behrendt, D.M.; Aberdeen, E.; Bonham-Carter, R.E.: Total anomalous pulmonary venous drainage. II. Spontaneous functional closure of interatrial communication after surgical correction in infancy. Circulation *66*: 357 (1972).

21 El-Said, G.; Mullins, C.E.; McNamara, D.G.: Management of total anomalous pulmonary venous return. Circulation *65*: 1240 (1972).

22 Mullins, C.E.; El-Said, G.M.; Neches, W.H.; Williams, R.L.; Vargo, T.A.; Nihill, M.R.; McNamara, D.G.: Balloon atrial septostomy for total anomalous pulmonary venous return. Br. Heart J. *35*: 752 (1973).

23 Drummond, W.H.; Gregory, G.A.; Heymann, M.A.; Phibbs, R.A.: The independent effects of hyperventilation, tolazoline and dopamine on infants with persistent pulmonary hypertension. Fetal and neonatal medicine. J.Pediat. *98*: 603 (1981).

24 Haworth, S.G.; Reid, L.: Structural study of pulmonary circulation and of heart in total anomalous pulmonary venous return in early infancy. Br.Heart J. *39*: 80–92 (1977).

25 Barratt-Boyes, B.G.: Techniques and results of treatment in total anomalous pulmonary venous connection; in Parenzan, Crupi, Graham, Patron, Congenital heart disease in the first 3 months of life, pp.461–471.

26 Shinebourne, E.A.; Del Torso, S.; Miller, G.A.H.; Jones, O.D.H.; Capuani, A.; Lincoln, C.: Total anomalous pulmonary venous drainage (TAPVRD); Medical aspects and surgical indications; in Parenzan, Crupi, Graham, Congenital heart disease in the first 3 months of life, pp.447–459 (Patron Editore, Bologna 1981).

27 Delisle, G.; Ando, M.; Calder, A.L.; Zuberbuhler, J.R.; Rochenmacher, S.; Alday, L.E.; Mangini, O.; Van Praagh, S.; Van Praagh, R.: Total anomalous venous connection: report of 93 autopsied cases with emphasis on diagnostic and surgical considerations. Am.Heart J. *91*: 99–122 (1976).

Peter B.Mansfield, MD, Department of Surgery, Children's Orthopedic Hospital and Medical Center, PO Box C5371, Seattle, WA 98105 (USA)

Mod. Probl. Paediat., vol. 22, pp. 110–115 (Karger, Basel 1983)

Complications of Mitral Valve Replacement in Children with Mitral Incompetence (Atrioventricular Canal Excluded)

J. V. Aubert[a], *L. Menicanti*[b], *J. M. Jarry*[a]

[a] CHU Timone-Hôpital d'Enfants, Marseille, France;
[b] Reparto di Chirurgia Pediatrica, Ospedale Civile, Vicenza, Italia

Mitral valve surgery in children is beset with many problems. In particular, for us, 89 % of our patients beeing of Algerian origin, and often living at some distance from large towns, make follow-up of anticoagulant treatment difficult or impossible. For this reason, between 1976 and 1979 we used biological prostheses in these children for mitral valve replacement, in order to avoid the need for anticoagulants on their return to Algeria.

This paper is a review of our medium-term results after 8 years of mitral valve replacements in order to identify areas for improvement in management. The number of cases in published series of mitral valve replacement in children is generally less than in the reports of similar surgery in adults. This is also true for our own series, and we therefore make no attempt at statistical analysis, which would be misleading in a series of only 47 operated cases. We have excluded from this study mitral valve replacement as part of the treatment of a complete atrioventricular canal, because it is impossible to evaluate the role of the mitral prosthesis in the immediate or medium-term complications of this complex malformation.

Patients and Methods

From January 1974 to January 1981, we operated on 47 children with mitral incompetence. 29 had a conservative operation, with repair of the mitral valve. 4 of these children were reoperated within 1 month for replacement of the valve after failure of the initial operation. We performed 50 mitral valve replacements, 43 primary procedures, 4 times after the failure of conservative surgery and 3 times to replace a failing biological prosthesis with a mechanical valve. This report describes the complications arising after these 50 operations in 47 children.

The mean age of the patients was 8.9 ± 4.1 years and their mean weight 20.2 ± 10.6 kg.

40 children had rheumatic mitral valve disease. In 4 cases we were unable to determine from the records the degree of cardiac insufficiency. 4 were in the NYHA group II and were operated on because of gross cardiomegaly with a cardiothoracic ratio greater than 70%, although functional signs were minimal. 23 children were in group III and 10 in group IV of the NYHA classification.

There were 4 cases of mitral incompetence complicating cardiomyopathy (1 glycogenosis, 1 familial cardiomyopathy). The mitral disease appeared to be greatly worsening the condition of these children, of which 3 were in NYHA group IV and 1 in group III.

There were 3 congenital malformations: 1 congenital mitral stenosis with mitral regurgitation, 1 triatrial heart with mitral reflux and severe left ventricular hypoplasia, and 1 case of Ebstein's syndrome with mitral reflux and atrioventricular discordance. These 3 children were all less than 4 years old at the time of surgery.

All operations were performed under extracorporeal circulation and moderate hypothermia, without aortic cross-clamping. The valve replacement was always carried out through a left auriculotomy, with a vent placed in the apex of the left ventricle. The valve was sewn in with interrupted U stitches. Valve replacements with a mechanical prosthesis were always started on anticoagulant therapy, with the exception of the first child given a St Jude valve, who developed a partial thrombosis of the valve 6 weeks later. Otherwise, immediate postoperative anticoagulation was with intravenous heparin, given whenever the clotting time was less than 10 min during 2 consecutive hours. Subsequently, Calciparine was given subcutaneously for the first 5 days postoperatively, followed by Coumadine if the coagulation profile on Calciparine was stable. Treatment with Digoxin was continued postoperatively in all cases.

Results

Mortality. 4 children died in the immediate postoperative period. 2 of these had complex congenital defects in addition to their mitral disease (triatrial heart with hypoplastic left ventricle and Ebstein's syndrome with atrioventricular discordance), these 2 children being 16 and 22 months old. Another child died as a result of obstruction of left ventricular outflow by his biological prosthesis, and the last death was due to acute left auricular thrombosis 6 h after implantation of a Starr-Edwards valve, before heparin treatment had been started.

Of the 43 children surviving the operation, 3 with cardiomyopathy died 3, 7 and 16 months later, from progression of the cardiomyopathy with a normally functioning prosthesis in all 3 cases. In the 40 survivors there were 6 late deaths. The 2 children with Bjork valves died suddenly from blockage of their valves in the closed position; 1 child 6 months after the operation, when he was perfectly well. The other had symptoms of valve dysfunction for an unknown period before his death, 9 years after the operation, in Algeria. Finally, 4 children died a mean of 2.4 years after the implantation of a biological prosthesis; 3 of these deaths were in Algeria and the fourth was a few hours after arriving in France with acute pulmonary edema. The overall mortality related to age is shown in table I.

Morbidity. Of 25 children with mechanical prostheses surviving the postoperative period, 19 continued their anticoagulant treatment in Algeria, with no thromboembolic or hemorragic complications. 2 discontinued anticoagulant therapy, of which 1 developed a hemiplegia 6 years after valve replacement. 4 have been lost to follow-up.

Failure of biological prostheses has been a much more serious problem, since 7 of the 20 children with these valves had this complication, and 4 died before corrective surgery could be undertaken. The 3 others arrived in Marseille in a moribund condition. 2 were operated on within 6 h of their admission to hospital and the third after 48 h, following correction of severe metabolic disorders. In all 3 cases a St Jude valve was used, with good results.

Discussion

Operative mortality was 8% (4 deaths in 50 operations) but in half it was due to severe congenital malformations, at the limits of present surgical technique. The other 2 deaths resulted 1 from an error in positioning the valve, with left ventricular outflow obstruction, and 1 probably as a result of an error in anticoagulation. We therefore feel that at least 2 of these 4 postoperative deaths could be avoided in the future.

Overall mortality appears to be related to age at the time of operation (table I), since 62% of those aged less than 4 years have died, compared with a mortality of 12% in those more than 8 years old.

3 deaths were due to the progression of cardiomyopathy, with no evidence of dysfunction of the valve prosthesis. This is a very controversial indication for valve replacement, because the operation has no effect on the progress of the myocardial disease, and can only prolong survival. It seems that, if these cases are considered for surgery on their secondary mitral valve disease, the operation should be carried out before they reach NYHA group IV. In fact we have operated on 3 cases of mitral incompetence secondary to cardiomyopathy in NYHA class III, performing mitral an-

Table I. Mortality

age, years	NB	Hospital deaths	Late deaths
0–4	8	2	3
4–8	10	0	3
8–12	21	1	2
12–16	8	1	0
Total	47	4	8

nuloplasty with, in 2 cases, repair of chordae and papillary muscle anomalies as well. These 3 children are well 15, 18 months and 3 years after operation, although 1 of them required a second operation 9 months later to implant a St Jude valve.

2 children died following the blockage in the closed position of their Bjork valves. We now believe that if it is necessary to insert a disc-type valve in a child the best choice is the St Jude valve, which has two discs and so avoids the complication of sudden death if a disc sticks, as the other usually continues to function. This was seen in 1 of our patients who developed partial thrombosis of his St Jude valve and whom we were able to reoperate 8 days later without difficulty. At present we have used a St Jude valve for mitral valve replacement on six occasions, and apart from one failure due to the lack of anticoagulant therapy, they are all working satisfactorily, 14–16 months postoperatively.

Provided that the patient can be regularly followed by a cardiologist there do not appear to be any particular problems in children with the anti-coagulant therapy which is essential with any type of mechanical prosthesis. The use of biological prostheses resulted in a very high rate of failure, this occurring in 7 of 20 cases (35 %) at a mean time of 3.4 $\pm$ 0.9 years after the operation. It is likely that the 4 who died without further surgery could have been saved if they had been well followed up, and readmitted to hospital on the appearance of a mitral murmur.

A further problem with both biological and mechanical prostheses is the growth of the child, which could lead to relative mitral stenosis, when it is necessary in young children, to implant a valve which is theoretically too small for an older child or an adult. Because of the relatively short follow-up in our series we have not yet encountered this problem.

Conclusion

Mitral valve replacement in children with mitral reflux is burdened with a large overall mortality, whereas the operative mortality should be less than 8 %. In our experience, late deaths are due largely to preexisting cardiomyopathy and to failure of biological prostheses. In addition, the mortality is very high in children of less than 4 years, for whom operation should only be considered if there is a definite risk to life in the short-term with medical treatment alone.

If the indications for valve replacement are absolute, whatever the age of the child, a mechanical prosthesis is to be preferred to a biological implant. These latter carry a considerable risk of serious complications during the first 5 years following implantation. In addition, it should be remembered that for an equivalent diameter there is a greather transvalvular gradient with biological than with mechanical prostheses, particularly with the St Jude valve. A further advantage of this type is that a St Jude number 25 valve, which is relatively small, poses no problems of stenosis until the child reaches a body surface area of 1.5 m^{-2}, or a body weight of about 40 kg. We believe that biological prostheses should only be used in patients older than 15 years in whom the risks of fibrosis and calcification are small, or in children who can be very closely followed to detect any malfunction of the valve at an early stage, leading in most cases to its replacement. In view of the near total absence of complications of anticoagulant therapy in children, we feel the use of biological prostheses to avoid this treatment does not confer any advantage. For this reason we have not used biological prostheses for mitral valve replacement in children since 1980.

When we implant a mechanical valve in a child our present choice is between a Starr-Edwards and a St Jude valve. The former has the advantage of having a considerable clinical follow-up, showing a minimal risk of complications, but it occupies a large volume, and can therefore only be used in children with an enlarged left ventricle. The St Jude valve does not have this problem, and has two discs, which should prevent sudden cardiac arrest, but we await long-term follow-up studies to show its real value.

In any case, in view of the problems encountered in children with mitral prostheses, we believe that mitral valve replacement should only be performed if it is impossible to repair the valve. We prefer conservative valve surgery, even if this leads to a valve replacement several years later, to a valve replacement at the outset. The only exception that we make to this rule is for those severely ill cachectic children in stage IV mitral reflux with metabolic and pulmonary complications for whom the only chance of sur-vival is with a valve replacement, to avoid any possibility of residual post-operative reflux, which would be fatal. This tendency towards a maximum of conservative surgery has seen our initial treatment of mitral incompetence in children change from valve replacements in 93 % of cases in 1974 to 50 % in 1981.

J. V. Aubert, MD, C. H. U. Timone – Hôpital d'Enfants, 27, Boulevard Jean Moulin, F-13005 Marseille (France)

Mod. Probl. Paediat., vol. 22, pp. 116–119 (Karger, Basel 1983)

Results of Cardiac Valve Replacement in 172 Children

B. Friedli, E. G. Benmimoun, J. C. Rouge, B. Faidutti

Clinique de Pédiatrie, Hôpital Cantonal Universitaire, Geneva, Switzerland

Severe valvular lesions, due to congenital malformations or following rheumatic heart disease, cannot always be repaired; thus, valve replacement by a prosthesis may become necessary even in children. We would like to report on a large series of children, many coming from third world countries, having undergone valve replacement in Geneva, and comment on the results of hemodynamic studies.

Clinical Data and Long-Term Follow-Up

Between 1969 and early 1980, 172 children underwent valve replacement in our hospital. Table I indicates the type of prosthesis used, and the site of implantation. The mitral valve was most often replaced, and mechanical valves were mostly used. The mean age at operation was 12 years, the range 2–17 years. Most patients had rheumatic valvular disease (161/172).

Hospital mortality was 5.8 %. The late mortality was 8.6 %, for a follow-up period of 1–10 years (mean 3.6 years). The main causes of late death were thromboembolism (5 cases), valve dysfunction (2 cases) and endocarditis (1 case).

The functional results are almost always excellent: most children lead normal, active lives and only 9 % remain digitalized. However, some complications occurred during the follow-up period of 1–10 years (table II). The main problem was thromboembolism, which occurred in 11 % (3 per 100 patient-years) despite anticoagulants or platelet-inhibiting drugs, which were taken by 75 % of the children. No thromboembolism occurred in children who had only aortic valve replacement.

Table I. Type and site of valve prosthesis

Type	Starr-Edwards	177
	Björk	26
	Hancock	6
Site	Mitral	117
	Aortic	18
	Tricuspid	1
	Double	34
	Triple	3

Table II. Complications

Thromboembolism (3/100 patient-years)		14
Died	5	
Residual lesions	4	
Complete recovery	5	
Prosthetic valve endocarditis		4
Died	1	
Cured	3	
Severe valve dysfunction		4
Died	1	
Reoperated	3	

Other complications were less frequent: endocarditis occurred in 4 cases and could be cured by medical treatment in 3. Valve dysfunction was seen in 4 cases (2 paravalvular leaks, 2 calcified Hancock prostheses).

'Outgrowing' has not been a problem in this series: indeed all mitral valves were replaced by adult size prostheses from age 4 years. This was possible because of the marked dilatation of the mitral valve annulus, usually occurring in mitral regurgitation. Only 3 pediatric size prostheses were used in this position (Starr-Edwards No. 1) and have not needed replacement by a larger one so far. In the aortic position, however, 16 pediatric size prostheses were implanted, which create some degree of stenosis: this has been well tolerated so far.

Hemodynamic Data and Left Ventricular Function

Hemodynamic study was undertaken in 44 children after mitral valve replacement, the indication for catheterization being either marked pul-

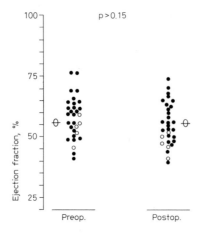

Fig. 1. LV ejection fraction before and after mitral valve replacement. There is no significant difference between means.

monary hypertension before surgery, or the suspicion of prosthetic valve dysfunction. The study took place 2–6 months (mean 3.9 months) after surgery. Preoperatively, pulmonary artery (PA) pressure was elevated, the mean PA pressure ranging from 18 to 75 mm Hg (mean 45.6 mm Hg). There was a marked decrease in PA pressure after surgery, with values ranging from 10 to 42, mean 23.4 mm Hg. This was partially due to a marked decrease in left atrial (pulmonary capillary wedge) pressure. However, pulmonary vascular (arteriolar) resistances (PVR) also dropped markedly: preoperatively, mean PVR was 590 dyn s cm^{-5}/m^2 (range 120–1,280), it dropped to a mean value of 282 dyn s cm^{-5}/m^2 (range 60–430). A return to normal resistance was observed in every case if the preoperative value was below 650 dynes cm^{-5}/m^2. Above this threshold, some degree of pulmonary hypertension usually persisted. In cases with residual mitral regurgitation (paravalvular leak), the pulmonary artery pressure and resistance usually remained at preoperative levels.

A residual gradient through the mitral prosthesis was often observed. This was slightly more important for the Hancock prostheses (mean 8.7 mm Hg) than for the Starr-Edwards prostheses (mean 6.9 mm Hg). Whereas one third of the children with Starr-Edwards prostheses have insignificant gradients (between 2 and 5 mm Hg), all children with Hancock prostheses have gradients above 5 mm Hg at rest.

Left ventricular (LV) volume and ejection fraction (EF) were measured angiographically before and after surgery in 30 patients. LV end-diastolic volume was elevated before surgery (83–379, mean 190 ml/m²). It decreased markedly after surgery to a mean of 103 ml/m² (range 55–250 ml/m²). A high postoperative LV volume was related to paravalvular leak in 3 patients and to significant aortic regurgitation in 1. Left ventricular EF (fig. 1) was often decreased preoperatively: the values ranged from 40 to 76%, mean 57%. Longstanding LV volume overload and the sequelae of rheumatic carditis are probably responsible for a depressed LV function seen in about one half of the cases. After surgery, there was no significant change in the mean EF, which was 56% (range 40–73%). No relation was found between EF and age of the patient. It must be recognized that a direct comparison of pre-operative and postoperative EF is not possible because of the different hemodynamic setting: by suppressing mitral regurgitation, a decrease in LV preload but an increase in afterload is obtained; this should result in a decrease of EF postoperatively, assuming myocardial contractility remains unchanged. We have not observed such a decrease, and this could be interpreted as an improved myocardial contractility postoperatively.

In conclusion, cardiac valve replacement can be achieved in children with a low hospital mortality and excellent results. Late postoperative complications, however, are not infrequent, the main problem being thromboembolism. Unfortunately, xenograft valves, with their low incidence of thromboembolism, are not suitable for children because of rapid calcification. Pulmonary hypertension, even of a severe degree, is not a contraindication for surgery, as it regresses postoperatively in most cases. Left ventricular dysfunction occurs frequently, due to the sequelae of rheumatic carditis and to longstanding volume overload. The current policy is to perform valve replacement only late in the disease, when grade III or IV heart failure is present; whether earlier valve replacement would prevent the problem of LV dysfunction cannot be answered from this study.

B. Friedli, MD, Clinique de Pédiatrie, Hôpital Cantonal Universitaire, CH-1200 Geneva (Switzerland)

Mod. Probl. Paediat., vol. 22, pp. 120–131 (Karger, Basel 1983)

Early and Late Results of Primary Repair
of Persistent Truncus Arteriosus

L. Parenzan, G. Crupi, R. Tiraboschi, M. Villani, P. Ferrazzi[1]

Department of Cardiac Surgery, Ospedali Riuniti, Bergamo, Italy

The natural history of patients born with persistent truncus arteriosus (PTA) is extremely poor. The majority of them die in congestive heart failure within the first year of life [1, 3] and at least one third of the survivors develop pulmonary vascular disease and are inoperable by the age of 4–5 years [4]. Early surgical treatment of these patients becomes mandatory after unsuccessful vigorous medical therapy. Primary repair represents the treatment of choice for patients with PTA [5, 10]. Although the hospital mortality rate in infants younger than 3 months of age remains considerably high [6, 10], the overall results compare favorably with those of pulmonary artery banding followed by late repair [6, 8]. Furthermore, pulmonary artery banding does not always prevent the development of pulmonary vascular disease [4, 11, 12] and may cause distorsion of the pulmonary arteries [11].

Primary repair can be achieved with significantly better results in older patients [6, 8, 10, 12, 13]. Long-term results of the survivors of truncus repair seem to be related to the preoperative presence of truncal valve regurgitation and elevated pulmonary vascular resistance [13]. Conduit replacement which is inevitable in patients undergoing repair in infancy does not seem to add to the initial surgical risk [5].

Clinical Material

From January 1974 through June 1981, 24 consecutive patients with PTA underwent primary repair at the department of Cardiac Surgery, Bergamo, Italy. No patient underwent pulmonary artery banding during that period. Their ages (table I) ranged from

---

[1] We are indebted to Miss *R. Pedrali* for the preparation of this manuscript.

Table I. Truncus arteriosus: age and weight

Age, months	Patients	Weight, kg (mean)
$\leq$ 3	6	3
> 3 $\leq$ 6	4	3.7
> 6 $\leq$ 12	6	5.3
> 12 $\leq$ 24	3	–
> 24	5	–
Total	24	–

30 days to 9 years (median age 17 months). 16 patients were younger than 1 year and their mean weight was 4 kg. 4 of the 6 infants younger than 3 months weighed less than 3 kg. Intractable heart failure was the indication for surgery in all 16 infants but one, a 7-month-old child with increased pulmonary vascular resistance (Rp/Rs = 0.63). Diagnosis of PTA was made at cardiac catheterization in each instance. The arterial oxygen saturation ranged from 70 to 98 % (mean 91 %) whereas the ratio between the pulmonary and systemic vascular resistance ranged from 0.25 to 0.63.

Definition of PTA was adapted from *Crupi* et al. [14]. Patients with PTA type IV of *Collett and Edwards* [15] are consequently not included in this study. The anatomic findings of PTA at the time of surgery are summarized in table II. Truncal valve regurgitation was present, as predicted at angiography, in 3 patients with grossly abnormal truncal valve. Stenosis of the right pulmonary artery necessitating extensive reconstruction was present in 2 patients. Associate anomalies (table III) included 2 cases of single coronary artery; right appendage juxtaposition with persistence of the left superior vena cava was present in one instance.

Surgical Technique

The operation was basically that described by *McGoon* et al. [16] in 1968. Separation of the pulmonary arteries is usually accomplished (fig. 1a) through a longitudinal incision in the anterior aspect of the arterial trunk. However, in two instances of PTA type III [15] it was necessary to transect the arterial trunk just above the origin of the pulmonary arteries. A generous ovoidal piece of truncal wall tissue containing the orifices of both pulmonary arteries, such as to make the anastomosis with the distal end of the valved conduit technically safer, is excised. Patch closure of the resulting truncal orifice has been carried out in the last 2 patients to avoid later supravalvular stenosis (see Late Results) and possible disturbance of the truncal valve mechanism. The distal conduit anastomosis (fig. 1b) is then constructed taking care to position the porcine valve ring as close as possible to the suture line. The ventricular septal defect (VSD; fig. 1c) is exposed through a longitudinal right ventriculotomy and closed by means of a Dacron-velour patch anchored in its superior circumference to the upper part of the ventriculotomy. The proximal end of the

Table II. Truncus arteriosus: anatomical findings

Truncus arteriosus	Patients	Truncal incompetence	Patients
Type I	10	severe	1
Type II	11	moderate	2
Type III	3		
		Pulmonary arteries	
Truncal valve		normal diameter	22
Bicuspid	2	RPA stenosis	2
Tricuspid	21		
Quadricuspid	1	Ventricular septal defect	
		TR-TR discontinuity	19
		TR-TR continuity	5

TR-TR = Truncal tricuspid

Table III. Truncus arteriosus: associated defects

Type	Patients
Single coronary artery	2
Right appendage juxtaposition	
and left superior vena cava	1
Atrial septal defect	23
Patent ductus arteriosus	2

conduit (fig. 1d) is anastomosed to the borders of the right ventriculotomy, suturing its posterior hemicircumference to the upper part of the VSD patch. Teflon strips are used to reinforce the anastomosis and to prevent bleeding from the suture line. The right ventricular outflow tract has always been reconstructed with an Hancock valved conduit. Until recently an oversized conduit which could be accommodated within the mediastinum without being compressed by the sternum was routinely used. Following *Ebert's* [5] experience we now prefer to use small-sized conduit in patients younger than 6 months in the belief that conduit replacement in this age group will be necessary regardless of its initial diameter. Furthermore, the use of a small conduit will allow for a smaller ventriculotomy with less impairment of the right ventricular function.

Surface-induced profound hypothermia with limited cardiopulmonary bypass and circulatory arrest remains our preferred technique of perfusion in patients younger than 1 year. However, profound hypothermia by core cooling and total circulatory arrest has been occasionally employed. Moderate hypothermia and cold potassium cardioplegia is routinely employed in older patients.

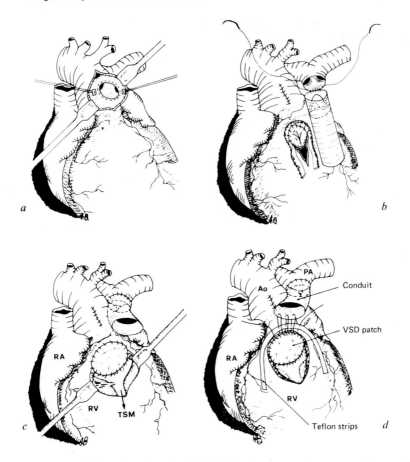

Fig. 1. Surgical repair. *a* Longitudinal incision in the anterior aspect of the arterial trunk in a case of PTA type I and identification of the origin of the pulmonary arteries (broken lines). *b* Detachment of the pulmonary arteries and construction of the distal conduit anastomosis. *c* Closure of the ventral septal defect (VSD). *d* Construction of the proximal conduit anastomosis. RA = Right atrium; RV = right ventricle; Ao = aorta; PA = pulmonary artery; TSM = Trabecula Septomarginalis.

Early Results

10 patients (table IV) died within 30 days of operation (41 %). 5 of the 6 infants younger than 3 months of life died whereas the mortality was appreciably lower (27 %) among the 18 older patients. The causes of early deaths are reported in table V.

Table IV. Truncus arteriosus: hospital deaths

Age, months	Patients	Deaths	%
≤ 3	6	5	83
> 3 ≤ 6	4	1	25
> 6 ≤ 12	6	2	33
> 12 ≤ 24	3	1	33
> 24	5	1	20
Total	24	10	41

Table V. Truncus arteriosus: causes of early death

Mode	Patients
Low cardiac output	5
Hemorrhage	2
Sepsis	2
Hemolysis	1
Total	10

Table VI. Truncus arteriosus: postoperative course – early survivors

Age, years	Patients	Intensive care unit days (mean)	Duration of mechanical ventilation days (mean)	Inotropic support
≤ 1	7	15	5	4/7
> 1	7	3.5	1	1/7

Table VII. Truncus arteriosus: late deaths

Patients	Age, months	Weight, kg	Postoperative p RV/LV	Interval from operation months	Cause
1	4	3.7	–	6	sudden
2	8	4.1	0.4		bronchopneumonia
3	10	6.6	0.6	2	sepsis

Table VIII. Truncus arteriosus: clinical status of late survivors

Patients	Median follow-up	Functional class			
	years	I	II	III	IV
11	4	7	4	–	–

Low cardiac output was the commonest cause of death. Intractable hemorrhage occurred in 2 patients: severe right pulmonary stenosis necessitating reconstruction with a Gore-Tex prosthesis was present in 1 case whereas prolonged preoperative mechanical ventilation was required in the other. 2 patients in whom the repair was considered entirely satisfactory (postoperative peak systolic RV/LV = 0.4) died of sepsis. The last patient with preoperative severe truncal valve regurgitation developed massive hemolysis due to trauma of the regurgitant blood stream against the VSD patch. This patient died 24 h after truncal valve replacement. Following this experience patients with preoperative truncal valve regurgitation have their VSD closed with a Dacron patch covered on its left side by autologous pericardium. Postoperative course (table VI) in the 14 early survivors showed that infants required a prolonged intubation and ventilation and a longer period of inotropic support and stay in intensive care unit as compared with older patients.

Late Results

3 patients (table VII) died within 6 months after repair. All were in good general condition at the discharge from hospital and 2 of them had satisfactory p RV/LV at the end of repair. Current information was available on all 11 survivors as of June 1980. Follow-up ranged from 8 months to 7 years after repair, with a median period of 4 years. The clinical status of late survivors according to NYHA[2] is reported in table VIII. Evidence of mild truncal regurgitation was present in 3 patients being clinically unchanged in degree in the 2 of them with preoperative regurgitation. 8 patients showed cardiac murmurs of increasing intensity suggestive of conduit stenosis. 1 patient with clinical evidence of porcine valve regurgitation underwent postoperative hemodynamic evaluation 5.6 years after repair performed at the

[2] New York Heart Association

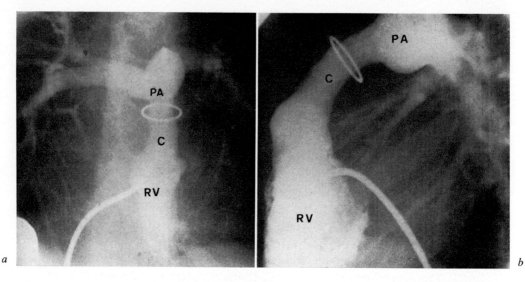

Fig. 2. Right ventricular injection: *a* anteroposterior and *b* lateral view showing mild narrowing of the conduit (C) lumen 5.6 years after implantation (Hancock No. 12). PA = Pulmonary artery; RV = right ventricle.

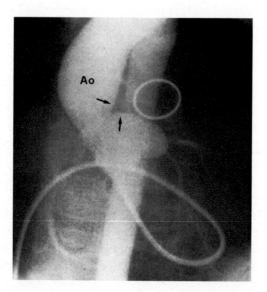

Fig. 3. Ascending aortography, anteroposterior view, showing mild 'supra-aortic stenosis' (double arrows) due to direct closure of the truncal defect after detachment of the pulmonary arteries. Ao = Aorta.

age of 5 months. Cardiac catheterization showed mild peak systolic gradients at the proximal conduit anastomosis (25 mm Hg) and at supraaortic level (15 mm Hg). Cineangiography revealed (fig. 2) severe porcine valve regurgitation with minimal narrowing of the conduit lumen. Supravalvular 'aortic' stenosis (fig. 3) was clearly related to direct closure of the defect resulting from detachment of the pulmonary arteries.

Discussion

Since the first successful report of *McGoon* et al. [16] in 1968 total repair for patients with PTA has become common. Yet the surgical risk varies significantly according to the age of patients at repair. Indeed, despite the outstanding results recently reported by *Ebert* [5] the hospital mortality rate in infancy remains consistently high, particularly when primary repair becomes necessary within the first 3 months of life [6, 10]. On the contrary the results achieved in older patients are far more satisfactory [13].

Unfortunately the majority of patients with PTA do require surgical management very early in life and other surgical options such as pulmonary artery banding followed by later repair seem to be associated with higher cumulative mortality [6, 8]. These considerations are confirmed by our own experience bearing in mind that no patients were denied operation because of young age, low weight, poor preoperative conditions or increased pulmonary vascular resistance. It is significant that low cardiac output was the cause of death only in the group of infants less than 3 months of age, 5 of whom died within 24 h after repair including 2 unable to be discontinued from bypass. We believe that our poor results are primarily related to both the young age and poor preoperative status of these patients all being in preoperative class IV [17].

Kirklin et al. [17], analyzing the total experience for open heart operation in infants under 3 months of age at Alabama University, found acute cardiac failure to be the most frequent cause of death. A multivariate logistic analysis of all preoperative factors indicated that young age and preoperative status were both significant incremental risk factors.

More encouraging are the results achieved in the remaining 10 older infants bearing in mind that 2 of the 3 hospital deaths in this age group were both due to sepsis in patients who had had an otherwise successful repair. Equally satisfactory are our results in patients older than 1 year with 2 hospital deaths both due to problems technically difficult to deal with, such as severe truncal valve regurgitation in one and diffuse stenosis of the right pulmonary artery in the other.

The late results of our 11 survivors have been satisfactory: most of them were in functional class I and none of them was receiving therapy. No patients have required conduit replacement although clinical evidence of progressive conduit stenosis was present in 8 of them. The 11 Hancock conduits were in place from 8 to 84 months (mean 48 months).

We believe that the long-term results of total repair of PTA are chiefly related to: (a) long-term performance of the Hancock conduits; (b) progression of pulmonary vascular disease; (c) long-term fate of the truncal valve.

Although the long-term performance of the porcine heterograft used for reconstruction of the right ventricular outflow tract in children remains uncertain [18], this seems to be related to the original size of the conduit at the time of implantation rather than to the performance of the porcine valve itself. *Ebert* [5] reported replacement of the original conduit within 3 years after surgery in 40% of 56 infants with PTA, all younger than 6 months of age. A 12-mm Hancock valved conduit had been implanted in most instances. Significantly different is the Mayo Clinic experience [19] with only 13 of 308 patients (4.2%) with right-sided valved conduit requiring conduit replacement at a mean interval of 50 months after implantation. Their mean age at surgery was 9 years and the diameter of the original Hancock conduit ranged from 16 to 25 mm (mean 20 mm). It is however very encouraging to see that the risk of changing the conduit to one of larger size would appear to be relatively small [5, 19].

Progression of pulmonary vascular disease can be very likely prevented by early repair before the age of 2 years [20]. However, a minority of infants with PTA have already elevated pulmonary vascular resistance at the time of repair. Whether primary repair even within the first 6 months of life would determine regression or even 'no progression' of the changes in the pulmonary vasculature remains purely speculative. Yet total repair, although associated with a significantly greater risk, seems to be indicated even in the presence of initially elevated pulmonary vascular resistance. Indeed, *Fuster* et al. [21] have shown 'no progression' of pulmonary vascular disease in a small number of patients who survived repair having initial pulmonary vascular resistance in excess of 7 U/m^2. Abnormalities of the truncal valve have been reported in several pathologic studies [14, 22, 23]. These include variation in size and number of the cusps, prolapse of the cusps and imperfectly formed commissures.

Nodular thickening of the cusps which is also a common finding at surgery is the more consistent abnormality. Nodularity seems to be related to stress [22] derived from the presence of a VSD and has a direct relationship with age. Whether early repair and reduction of flow across the truncal valve will reduce the likelihood of the development or progression of truncal valve incompetence is as yet undetermined. Interestingly, however, truncal valve regurgitation was present in 55 of 92 patients (median age 7.3 years) reported by *Marcelletti* et al. [13], being severe enough to require intraoperative treatment in 23 cases. On the contrary, only 14 of 56 infants reported by *Ebert* [5] had some degree of truncal valve regurgitation and none of them required treatment. Late results after repair of PTA have been related to the preoperative presence of truncal valve regurgitation [13]. These are significantly worse for patients with severe regurgitation as compared with no or only mild regurgitation.

In conclusion, we believe that early repair is the treatment of choice in all infants with PTA who are in congestive heart failure refractory to aggressive medical treatment. Elective repair is recommended before the age of 2 years to minimize the risk of pulmonary vascular disease developing either before or after correction. Furthermore, early repair by reducing the flow across the truncal valve will hopefully allow for a better performance of the valve itself. Long-term follow-up of the survivors of truncus repair has been satisfactory in the absence of significant truncal valve regurgitation and elevated pulmonary vascular resistances. However, further data are awaited on the long-term follow-up of patients surviving repair in infancy before any conclusion can be attempted.

References

1   Tandon, R.; Hauck, A.T.; Nadas, A.S.: Persistent truncus arteriosus. A clinical, hemodynamic and autopsy study of nineteen cases. Circulation *28:* 1050–1060 (1963).
2   Victorica, B.E.; Krovetz, L.J.; Elliot, L.P.; Van Mierop, L.H.S.; Bartley, T.D.; Gessner, I.H.; Schiebler, G.L.: Persistent truncus arteriosus in infancy. A study of 14 cases. Am.Heart J.*77:* 13–25 (1969).
3   Van Praagh, R.; Van Praagh, S.: The anatomy of common aortico-pulmonary trunk (truncus arteriosus communis) and its embryologic implications: a study of 57 necropsy cases. Am.J.Cardiol.*16:* 406–425 (1965).
4   Mair, D.D.; Ritter, D.G.; Davis, G.D.; Wallace, R.B.; Danielson, G.R.; McGoon, D.G.: Selection of patients with truncus arteriosus for surgical correction. Circulation *49:* 144–151 (1974).
5   Ebert, P.A.: Truncus arteriosus: size of the problem and results; in Parenzan, Crupi,

Graham, Congenital heart disease in the first 3 months of life. Medical and surgical aspects, pp.439–445 (Patron Editore, Bologna 1981).

6   Musumeci, F.; Piccoli, G.; Dickinson, D.F.; Hamilton, D.I.: Surgical experience with persistent truncus arteriosus in symptomatic infants under 1 year of age. Report of 13 consecutive cases. Br. Heart J. *46:* 179–185 (1981).

7   Stark, J.; Gandhi, D.; DeLeval, M.; Macartney, F.; Taylor, J.F.N.: Surgical treatment of persistent truncus arteriosus in the first year of life. Br. Heart J. *40:* 1280–1287 (1978).

8   Appelbaum, A.; Bargeron, J.H., Jr.; Pacifico, A.D.; Kirklin, J.W.: Surgical treatment of truncus arteriosus with emphasis on infants and small children. J. thorac. cardiovasc. Surg. *71:* 436–440 (1976).

9   Barratt-Boyes, B.G.: Complete correction of cardiovascular malformations in the first two years of life using profound hypothermia; in Barratt-Boyes, Neutze, Harris, Heart disease in infancy. Diagnosis and surgical treatment, pp.25–36, (Churchill-Livingstone, London 1973).

10 Parenzan, L.; Crupi, G.; Alfieri, O.; Bianchi, T.; Vanini, V.; Locatelli, G.; Tiraboschi, R.; Di Benedetto, G.; Villani, M.; Annecchino, F.P.; Ferrazzi, P.: Surgical repair of persistent truncus arteriosus in infancy. Thorac. cardiovasc. surg. *28:* 18–20 (1980).

11 McFaul, R.C.; Mair, D.D.; Feldt, R.H.; Ritter, D.G.; McGoon, D.G.: Truncus arteriosus and previous pulmonary artery banding: clinical and hemodynamic assessment. Am. J. Cardiol. *38:* 626–632 (1976).

12 Poirier, R.A.; Berman, M.A.; Stansel, H.C., Jr.: Current status of the surgical treatment of truncus arteriosus. J. thorac. cardiovasc. Surg. *69:* 169–182 (1975).

13 Marcelletti, C.; McGoon, D.G.; Danielson, G.K.; Wallace, R.B.; Mair, D.D.: Early and late results of surgical repair of truncus arteriosus. Circulation *55:* 636–641 (1977).

14 Crupi, G.; Macartney, F.J.; Anderson, R.H.: Persistent truncus arteriosus. A study of 66 autopsy cases with special reference to definition and morphogenesis. Am. J. Cardiol. *40:* 569–578 (1977).

15 Collett, R.W.; Edwards, J.E.: Persistent truncus ateriosus: a classification according to anatomic types. Surg. Clins. N. Am. *29:* 1245 (1949).

16 McGoon, D.C.; Rastelli, G.C.; Ongley, P.A.: An operation for the correction of truncus arteriosus. J. Am. med. Ass. *205:* 69–73 (1968).

17 Kirklin, J.K.; Blackstone, E.H.; Kirklin, J.W.; Stewart, R.W.; Pacifico, A.D.; Bargeron, L.M.: Management of the cardiac subsystem after cardiac surgery; in Parenzan, Crupi, Graham, Congenital heart disease in the first 3 months of life. Medical and surgical aspects, pp.33–41 (Patron Editore, Bologna 1981).

18 Bisset, G.S.; Schwartz, D.C.; Benzing, G.; Helmsworth, J.; Kaplan, S.: Late results of reconstruction of the right ventricular outflow tract with valved external conduits in children (Abstract). Am. J. Cardiol. *45:* 448 (1980).

19 Agarwal, K.C.; Edwards, W.D.; Feldt, R.H.; Danielson, G.K.; Puga, F.J.; McGoon, D.C.: Clinico-pathologic correlates of obstructed right-sided porcine-valved extracardiac conduits. J. thorac. cardiovasc. Surg. *81:* 591–601 (1980).

20 Dushine, J.W.; Kirklin, J.W.: Late results of the repair of ventricular septal defect on pulmonary vascular disease; in Kirklin, Advances in cardiovascular surgery, p.9 (Grune & Stratton, New York 1973).

21   Fuster, V.; Mair, D.D.; Ritter, D.G.; McGoon, D.C.: Truncus arteriosus with pulmonary vascular obstructive disease. Medical vs surgical management (Abstract). Am.J.Cardiol.*45:* 450 (1980).

22   Becker, A.E.; Becker, H.J.; Edwards, J.E.: Pathology of the semilunar valve in persistent truncus arteriosus. J.thorac.cardiovasc.Surg.*62:* 16–26 (1971).

23   Gelband, H.; Van Meter, S.; Gersony, W.M.: Truncal valve abnormalities in infants with persistent truncus arteriosus. A clinico-pathologic study. Circulation *45:* 397–403 (1972).

L.Parenzan, MD, Department of Cardiac Surgery, Ospedali Riuniti,
I-24100 Bergamo (Italy)

Mod. Probl. Paediat., vol. 22, pp. 132–138 (Karger, Basel 1983)

Surgery for Complete Form of Atrioventricular Canal: Early and Late Results

Gordon K. Danielson

Department of Surgery, Mayo Foundation, Mayo Clinic, Mayo Graduate School of Medicine, Rochester, Minn., USA

Successful correction of the complete form of atrioventricular (AV) canal is now readily achievable. The most challenging technical feature of this anomaly is the associated mitral valvular deformity. From a surgical standpoint, we have found it helpful to classify AV canal according to *Rastelli's* original types, based on the anatomy of the common anterior leaflet [1, 2].

Repair is conducted with cardiopulmonary bypass combined with hypothermia at 20°C. Cold potassium cardioplegic solution is infused every 30 min and topical hypothermia is added to keep the myocardial temperature below 20°C. The repair is performed through a right atriotomy. Ideal exposure is gained by mobilization of the caval cannulae as shown in figure 1a. After the anatomy of the anterior and posterior common leaflets is determined, the initial step in the repair is the approximation of their mitral components with a few interrupted sutures. If the anterior common leaflet is type A and incompletely divided, or is type C, the leaflet is incised to the anulus at the junction of mitral and tricuspid portions. A similar incision of the posterior common leaflet may be required, as shown by the dotted line, in patients with an interventricular communication beneath this leaflet.

A single prosthetic patch is fashioned in an oval shape and of a size comparable to that of the overall ventricular and atrial septal defect (fig. 1b). The inferior portion of the patch is sutured with interrupted sutures to the right side of the ventricular septum. All of the sutures are placed prior to lowering the patch into position.

The mitral and tricuspid margins of the naturally divided or incised anterior common leaflet are then sutured to the patch with interrupted horizontal mattress sutures at a level which corresponds to the plane of the normal mitral and tricuspid anuli (fig. 1c). The incised or naturally divided posterior common leaflet is attached to the patch in a similar manner.

In those cases in which the posterior common leaflet is attached to the interventricular septum by a membrane or fused chordae, the patch shape is altered so it can be sewn directly to the atrial surface of the leaflet (fig. 1d).

The valve is then tested by injecting saline forcefully into the left ventricle. Additional sutures are added where required. If a central leak is present, the valve anulus is narrowed by a double anuloplasty technique. The final step in the repair is closure of the atrial portion of the septal defect by suturing the most cephalad portion of the patch to the rim of the atrial septum (fig. 1e). In the presence of associated pulmonary stenosis, valvotomy and infundibular resection are performed as indicated.

A variation of the repair in which individual patches are used to close the atrial and ventricular septal defects has been employed in some circumstances. This two-patch technique has theoretical advantages for repair in infants, as there is no shortening of leaflet substance which occurs when divided leaflets are attached to a single patch. Another variation, which is designed to decrease the risk of heart block, employs an extension of the atrial portion of the patch which is sutured around the coronary sinus, thus avoiding crossing the plane of the conduction bundle during closure of the atrial septal defect.

We believe that an integral part of the operation for atrioventricular canal is the performance of intraoperative double sampling indocyanine dye curves. Withdrawal catheters are passed off from the operating table and connected to dual densitometers. The curves are performed by injecting into the left ventricle and sampling simultaneously in the left atrium and ascending aorta. The amount of early-appearing dye in the left atrium quantitates the degree of mitral regurgitation. If severe regurgitation is demonstrated (regurgitant fraction greater than 20–25%), bypass is resumed, the left atrium is entered, and the repair is revised or the valve is replaced with a prosthesis.

Associated mitral valvular deformities can pose special technical problems in the repair of both partial and complete atrioventricular canal. In our series of 241 patients undergoing operation, 20 (8.3%) had severe deformities of the mitral valve including parachute mitral valve (single papillary muscle) (2.1%), double orifice mitral valve (4.1%), and miscellaneous defects such as double clefts (2.1%).

Our surgical mortality for complete repair of AV canal prior to June 1963 was 60%. The standardized operation described earlier was then devel-

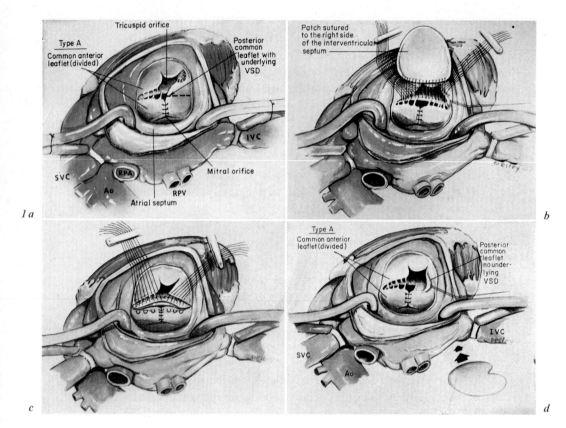

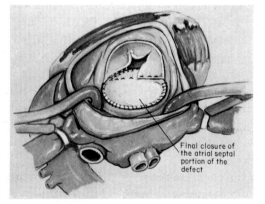

oped and the mortality dropped to 7 % in the next 27 patients. However, all 27 patients were 3 years of age or older. Younger patients were banded, with inconsistent results. Subsequently, we have accepted symptomatic patients of any age for repair [3].

There were 150 patients undergoing repair of complete AV canal between 1963 and September 1980 (table I). The total hospital (30 day) mortality was 14 %. The mortality for patients aged 3 years to 23 years was only 4.7 %. It is interesting that the mortality in patients less than 12 months of age was actually less than in the 1- to 2-year group. This is probably related to the development of pulmonary vascular obstructive disease in the older group and to our acceptance of borderline candidates for operation in order to not exclude those patients with pulmonary hypertension who might achieve an excellent long-term result following repair of their defect.

Only 1 patient required mitral valve replacement at the time of repair.

96 survivors of reparative operation between 1967 and 1978 were followed for 2–12 years (mean 5.1 years). There were 4 late deaths. The New York Heart Association functional classifications of the survivors were: class I, 70 %; class II, 25 %, and class III, 1 %.

Postoperative cardiac catheterizations were performed in 23 patients, most of whom were symptomatic. Mitral incompetence was assessed as severe in 1, moderate in 5, mild in 12, and absent in 5. 6 patients (6 %) required mitral valve replacement during the follow-up interval.

23 patients had catheterization data before operation and at follow-up 1–8 years later (mean 4.2 years) which allowed calculation of pulmonary arteriolar resistance (table II). The most favorable group had resistances less than 5 U · m².

There were 208 patients with complete AV canal who were evaluated at our institution between 1960 and 1978 [4]. 46 (22 %) had pulmonary arteriolar resistances equal to or greater than 5 U · m². 15 of the 46 (33 %) had Down's syndrome whereas only 17 % of the overall group were Down patients. This finding supports the clinical impression that patients with

---

Fig. 1. Repair of complete AV canal, type A. *a* Repair of mitral valve. *b* Insertion of oval prosthetic patch the size of the combined atrial and ventricular septal defects. All sutures to the right side of the septum are placed before the patch is lowered into position. *c* The patch is sutured to the leaflets at a level that corresponds to that of the normal mitral and tricuspid anuli. *d* If the posterior common leaflet is attached to the interventricular septum by a membrane or fused chordae, a patch of different shape is sewn to the atrial surface of the leaflet. *e* The final step. The most cephaled portion of the patch is sutured to the rim of the atrial septum [from ref. 2].

Table I. Surgical repair of complete atrioventricular canal: 1963 to September 1980

Age	Patients	Mortality number	%
< 12 months	21	5	23.8
1–2 years	44	12	27.3
3–23 years	85	4	4.7
Total	150	21	14.0

Table II. Complete atrioventricular canal

Pulmonary arteriolar resistance

preoperative U · m²	number of patients	at follow-up (1–8 years) decreased or same	increased
< 5	15	13	2
5–10	6	3	3
> 10	2	0	2
Total	23	16	7

Down's syndrome are more prone to develop pulmonary vascular obstructive disease. The ages of the 46 patients ranged from 5 months to 32 years (mean 6.5 years).

Follow-up ranged from 1 to 21 years, with a mean of 10 years. Of the 33 patients with pulmonary arteriolar resistance 5–13 $U \cdot m^2$, 18 were treated medically and 15 surgically. All 13 patients with resistance of 14 $U \cdot m^2$ or over were treated medically. The results are shown in table III. The only patients who improved were those treated surgically (54% of the surgical group improved), whereas all of the medically treated patients deteriorated or died.

In our experience in a follow-up of over 20 years, over 90% of patients with a preoperative pulmonary arteriolar resistance less than 5 $U \cdot m^2$ have had a good late result. In contrast to this, only 50–60% of patients with a resistance of 5 $U \cdot m^2$ or greater have had a good late result.

A relationship has been found between the pulmonary arterial oxygen saturation and the results in the surgical patients with pulmonary arteriolar resistance elevated to 5–13 $U \cdot m^2$. If the saturation is 85% or greater, the late results are generally good, whereas 80% of patients with a saturation of 84% or less have deteriorated or died at follow-up.

Table III. Repair of complete atrioventricular canal with PVOD

| Clinical status at follow-up | Rpa = 5–13 U · m² | | | | Rpa ≥ 14 U · m²: | |
| | surgical | | medical | | medical | |
	number	%	number	%	number	%
Improvement	8	54	0	–	0	–
Deterioration	2	13	11	61	7	54
Mortality	5	33	7	39	6	46
Total	15	100	18	100	13	100

PVOD = Pulmonary vascular obstructive disease: Rpa = pulmonary arteriolar resistance.

These data have led us to suggest the following criteria of operability: (1) If the pulmonary arteriolar resistance is less than 5 U, the operative risk is small and the late results are good. (2) If the pulmonary arteriolar resistance is 5–13 U · m² (total pulmonary resistance 7–14 U · m²), the pulmonary arterial oxygen saturation is determined. If the saturation is 85 % or greater, surgical treatment is advised. If the saturation is less than 85 %, surgical treatment is not advised except in patients 1–2 years of age (infants are excluded, as there is a greater chance for regression of pulmonary vascular obstructive disease after repair in patients 2 years of age or younger). (3) If the pulmonary arteriolar resistance is 14 U · m² or greater (total pulmonary resistance 15 U · m² or greater), surgical treatment is not advised.

Mention should also be made of repair of complete AV canal associated with additional complex congenital cardiac lesions. Until recently, attempted repairs usually resulted in an unsuccessful outcome. Several recent cases of successful repair of complicated forms of complete AV canal give encouragement to the present capability to accomplish repair of such complex lesions, even in the infant group. One example is given in the report of a 2-year-old girl who underwent repair of a complete AV canal associated with isolated dextrocardia, common atrium, total anomalous systemic venous return to a left superior vena cava, and double orifice mitral valve [5].

Complete AV canal associated with either common ventricle (type IC) or giant ventricular septal defect and insufficiency of both AV valves requiring valve replacement has also been successfully accomplished [6].

Another example of complete AV canal associated with other complex cardiac anomalies is given in the report of a 6-year-old girl who had the combination of complete AV canal, double outlet right ventricle, and atrioventricular discordance [7]. In addition, there was dextrocardia, common atrium, bilateral superior venae cavae, and pulmonary stenosis. A previous ascending aorta-left pulmonary artery (Waterston) anastomosis had been performed and subsequently a left Blalock anastomosis was constructed. Repair was accomplished by ligation of the left subclavian artery, take-down of the Waterston anastomosis with pericardial patch enlargement of the left pulmonary artery, repair of the AV canal in the classical fashion, and insertion of a valved conduit between the pulmonary ventricle and the pulmonary artery. She represents the first successful repair of this anomaly and is doing well 5 years later.

In summary, complete atrioventricular canal can now be repaired satisfactorily at all ages. The most challenging technical feature of this anomaly is the associated mitral valvular deformity. In most circumstances, we prefer primary repair in infancy rather than a two-stage procedure. Many complex forms of complete atrioventricular canal are also now amenable to total correction.

References

1   Rastelli, G.C.; Kirklin, J.W.; Titus, J.L.: Anatomic observations on complete form of persistent common atrioventricular canal with special reference to atrioventricular valves. Mayo Clin. Proc. *41:* 296 (1966).
2   McMullan, M.H.; Wallace, R.B.; Weidman, W.H.; McGoon, D.C.: Surgical treatment of complete atrioventricular canal. Surgery, St. Louis *72:* 905 (1972).
3   McGoon, D.C.; McMullan, M.H.; Mair, D.D.; Danielson, G.K.: Correction of complete atrioventricular canal in infants. Mayo Clin. Proc. *48:* 769 (1973).
4   Fuster, V.; Feldt, R.H.; Ritter, D.G.; McGoon, D.C.: Complete atrioventricular canal defect with pulmonary vascular obstructive disease – medical versus surgical management. Proc. Wld Congr. Paediatric Cardiology, London 1980, abstract No. 008.
5   Danielson, G.K.; McMullan, M.H.; Kinsley, R.H.; DuShane, J.W.: Successful repair of complete atrioventricular canal associated with dextroversion, common atrium, and total anomalous systemic venous return. J. thorac. cardiovasc. Surg. *66:* 817 (1973).
6   Danielson, G.K.; Giuliani, E.R.; Ritter, D.G.: Successful repair of common ventricle associated with complete atrioventricular canal. J. thorac. cardiovasc. Surg. *67:* 152 (1974).
7   Danielson, G.K.; Tabry, I.F.; Ritter, D.G.; Maloney, J.D.: Successful repair of double-outlet right ventricle, complete atrioventricular canal, and atrioventricular discordance associated with dextrocardia and pulmonary stenosis. J. thorac. cardiovasc. Surg. *76:* 710 (1978).

Gordon K. Danielson, MD, Department of Surgery, Mayo Foundation, Mayo Clinic, Mayo Graduate School of Medicine, Rochester, MN 55905 (USA)

Mod. Probl. Paediat., vol. 22, pp. 139–151 (Karger, Basel 1983)

Tetralogy of Fallot: Principles of Surgical Management

James K. Kirklin, Albert D. Pacifico, John W. Kirklin

Department of Surgery, Division of Cardiovascular and Thoracic Surgery, University of Alabama in Birmingham, University Station, Birmingham, Ala., USA

Natural History and Late Results

The natural history of tetralogy of Fallot without surgical treatment is poor. Data from *Bertranou* et al. [1] indicated that 30 % of surgically untreated patients are dead by 1 year of age and 50 % by 5 years of age. After about 5 years, the proportion of surviving patients decreases at a nearly steady rate. The most common cause of death is hypoxia, and less common causes include pulmonary thrombosis, pulmonary hemorrhage, cerebral thrombosis, and brain abscess. With this very poor natural history, nearly all patients with tetralogy of Fallot should be considered for surgical intervention.

In sharp contrast to the natural history of tetralogy of Fallot, the late results after complete repair are quite fantastic. It is amazing that even from the early days of open heart surgery at the Mayo Clinic, patients who survived corrective operation for tetralogy had a superb long-term result [2]. An actuarial analysis of the 396 hospital survivors after repair of tetralogy of Fallot at the Mayo Clinic between 1955 and 1965 indicates that over 90 % of the hospital survivors were alive 19 years later. Most of the deaths occurred during the first 5 years after operation and were most likely related to incomplete repairs during the very early years of open heart surgery.

Analysis of survivors after operations performed during the subsequent decade at the University of Alabama indicates similar long-term results [3]. 96 % of patients leaving the hospital were alive 8 years later, a result not significantly different from the early Mayo Clinic experience. It will thus be very difficult to improve upon these long-term results despite our continued advances in preoperative diagnosis, intraoperative techniques, and postoperative management.

Analysis of the Mayo Clinic and University of Alabama experience has identified some of the incremental risk factors for premature death after correction of tetralogy [3]. A high post-repair right ventricular pressure was an incremental risk factor in both series. Although not conclusively shown, a high post-repair right ventricular pressure probably becomes important when the ratio of right to left ventricular pressure exceeds about 0.7. A large residual ventricular septal defect (VSD) with a pulmonary to systemic blood flow ratio greater than 2 increased the risk of premature death. A previous Potts anastomosis was an incremental risk factor in both series. Although not demonstrable in the Mayo Clinic experience, the University of Alabama data suggested that older age at operation, possibly over about 5 years of age, may decrease long-term survival. Transannular patching, a previous Blalock or Waterston shunt, and bifasicular block on electrocardiogram were not associated with premature death. It is our belief, however, that trans-annular patching may be associated with an increase risk of premature death during the second 20 years of follow-up if it is accompanied by progressive cardiomegaly.

The deleterious effect of a residual VSD after repair is emphasized by a report from *Rocchini* et al. [4] from Boston. Among 58 patients with a residual VSD 1–12 years after repair of tetralogy, congestive heart failure was present in all patients with a pulmonary to systemic blood flow ratio greater than 2.0.

A detailed study of exercise tolerance in 135 patients a mean of 7 years after complete repair of tetralogy by *Wessel* et al. [5] identified certain variables which adversely affect late exercise tolerance (table I). The presence of a large *residual VSD* was associated with only 67 % of normal exercise tolerance. Patients undergoing *primary repair* had nearly normal exercise tolerance, which was not significantly different from *two-stage repair* with a *Blalock-Taussig* shunt. A *previous Potts* shunt, however, significantly reduced exercise tolerance compared with primary repair. If patients with a residual VSD and with pulmonary valve incompetence were excluded, there was no difference in exercise tolerance between patients with a peak right ventricular pressure above 50 mm Hg and a peak pressure below 50 mm Hg. Only a few patients, however, had peak pressures greater than 70 mm Hg.

The presence of *post-repair pulmonary valve incompetence* was associated with a significant reduction in exercise even in the presence of low right ventricular pressures. When pulmonary valve incompetence is combined with high right ventricular pressures, there was even greater reduction in exercise tolerance. The late effects of transannular patching are especially

Table I. Duration of exercise (min) after repair of tetralogy of Fallot [5]

Residual VSD vs no residual VSD	$p < 0.001$
Primary vs subclavian-pulmonary shunts	N.S.
Primary vs potts	$p < 0.05$
$P_{RV} \leqslant 50$ vs $P_{RV} > 50$, no PI (no VSD)	N.S.
$P_{RV} \leqslant 50$ no PI vs with PI (no VSD)	$p < 0.05$
$P_{RV} > 50$ no PI vs with PI (no VSD)	$p < 0.02$

VSD = Ventricular septal defect; PI = pulmonary incompetence;
N.S. = non-significant.

Table II. Lessons from late studies in tetralogy of Fallot

Long-term prognosis is *excellent*, so make the *patient* a *hospital survivor* of *complete repair*,
   and:

Avoid a Potts anastomosis for initial palliation
Avoid delaying repair too long (? > 5 years of age)
Avoid leaving a residual VSD
Avoid a high late post-repair $P_{RV/LV}$ (? > 0.7)
Avoid a transannular patch 'unless necessary'

VSD = Ventricular septal defect; $P_{RV/LV}$ = ratio of peak pressure in right ventricle to
that in left ventricle.

interesting. Patients with a *transannular patch* and a *normal heart size* had
nearly normal exercise tolerance. In contrast, patients with a *transannular
patch* and *cardiomegaly* as judged by the cardiothoracic ratio on chest
roentgenogram had a significantly lower exercise tolerance. Although we do
not know the exact incidence of late cardiomegaly associated with transannular patching, it seems likely that the incidence will gradually increase
with time.

   In summary then, factors which jeopardize late postoperative exercise
capacity and/or long term survival include a previous Potts anastomosis,
older age at time of repair, residual VSD, high post-repair right ventricular
pressures (probably greater than 70 mm Hg), and a transannular patch when
combined with cardiomegaly.

   Certain lessons can be gained from these long-term studies of function
and survival after complete repair of tetralogy of Fallot (table II). We must
remember that if the patient survives the hospital period after complete repair, the long-term prognosis is excellent. In addition, we should not use a

Table III. Possible contraindications to complete repair in tetralogy

Young age
High predicted post-repair $P_{RV/LV}$
Need for transannular patch
Anomalous anterior descending artery
Major associated lesions

Potts anastomosis for initial palliation. The repair should not be delayed too long, probably greater than 5 years of age. We should avoid leaving a residual VSD and a high late post-repair PRV/LV ratio (ratio of peak pressure in the right ventricle compared to that in the left ventricle), probably greater than 0.7. A transannular patch should not be used 'unless it is necessary'. Specific indications for transannular patching will be discussed, and are known to vary considerably among surgeons.

Current Controversies in Tetralogy

Contraindications to Primary Repair
From the time of the first intracardiac repair of tetralogy by *Lillehei* et al. [6] in 1954, no one seriously entertained a policy of routine primary correction of tetralogy of Fallot in infancy until *Barratt-Boyes and Neutze* [7] in 1973 reported on 25 infants with symptomatic tetralogy of Fallot. Primary repair was accomplished using techniques of surface cooling, deep hypothermia, total circulatory arrest, and limited cardiopulmonary bypass. The operative mortality was 4%.—

Since then, many surgical groups have reported good results for primary repair of tetralogy in infancy. It is important to remember, however, that these series do not represent a policy of routine primary repair in infancy. Although there is certainly not uniform agreement, each surgeon has certain important contraindications in his own mind to complete repair in early infancy (table III).

Although young age was once a contraindication to complete repair, few surgeons would elect an initial palliative operation on the basis of young age alone. If the predicted post-repair PRV/LV, even with the use of a transannular patch, is greater than about 0.8–1.0, repair is probably not advisable. In some institutions, the need for transannular patching in very young or very small infants is a contraindication to primary repair. Early repair may not be advisable in the presence of an anomalous anterior descending coronary artery arising from the right coronary artery and passing across the right ventricular outflow area, since this may necessitate the use of an external conduit. For many, the presence of major associated lesions is a relative contraindication to early primary repair.

Perhaps the most complex of these problems is the prediction of the post-repair P RV/LV preoperatively. We know that in certain patients severe right ventricular hypertension will persist even after satisfactory infundibular resection and pulmonary valvotomy. Such patients may have a small pulmonary annulus, and in this situation a transannular patch may be required. A few patients may continue to have a high post-repair PRV/LV even in the presence of an adequate transannular patch combined with complete relief of infundibular obstruction. Such patients may have unrelieved obstruction of the orifice of the right or the left pulmonary artery, abnormalities in the distribution of the pulmonary arterial system (arborization anomalies), or hypoplastic right or left pulmonary arteries.

We can quantite the effect of each of these areas of obstruction by applying nomograms which have been generated by *Rowlatt* et al. [8] as well as workers at the University of Alabama. In 1963, these authors presented regression equations based on measurements of 75 autopsy specimens from which the average normal annulus circumference and its standard deviation could be calculated according to body surface area. Thus, we can determine a so-called Z value which is equal to the number of standard deviations by which the actual ring circumference deviates from the mean normal circumference.

$$Z = \frac{\text{actual ring circumference} - \text{mean normal circumference.}}{\text{standard deviation of normal circumference}}$$

The size of the pulmonary valve ring in each individual patient is calculated as its degree of normality (Z), the number of standard deviations by which actual ring circumference deviates from the mean normal circumference [16].

In order to predict the post-repair P RV/LV, it is necessary to assess certain anatomic features angiographically, and relate these to the normal. If there is complete relief of infundibular obstruction and a transannular patch is utilized, the post-repair PRV/LV is generally related to the sum of the diameters of the right and left pulmonary arteries divided by the diameter of the descending aorta [9] (fig. 1). When this ratio is greater than

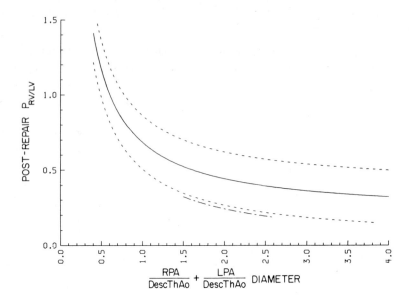

Fig.1. Nomogram for determination of post-repair $P_{RV/LV}$ based on angiographically determined size of right and left pulmonary arteries and diameter of descending thoracic aorta when a transannular patch or valved external conduit is used. Dashed lines enclose the 70% confidence limits [from ref. 9].

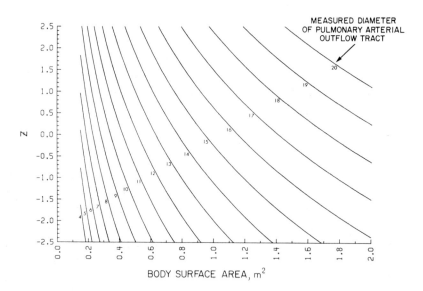

Fig.2. Nomogram for the determination of the Z-value for circumference for the individual patient from measurements at operation of the internal diameter (mm) of the narrowest part of the pulmonary arterial outflow tract and body surface area [ref. 10].

about 1.5, the post-repair PRV/LV will be less than 0.5, but when this ratio falls below 1.5, the expected post-repair PRV/LV begins to rise rapidly.

We must also carefully evaluate the pulmonary annulus preoperatively. In figure 2, nomograms are displayed for various diameters of the pulmonary artery outflow tract [10]. Thus, a Z value can be generated for each size of the pulmonary outflow tract if the body surface area is known. When a transannular patch is not used in the repair, a further increase in the post-repair PRV/LV usually results depending on the size of the pulmonary annulus. In figure 3, we see a nomogram of the relationship between the Z value as determined by the size of the pulmonary annulus and the body surface area, and the resultant further increase in post-repair PRV/LV if *no transannular patch* is used [9]. In general, if the ratio of right and left pulmonary arteries to the descending thoracic aorta is greater than about 1.5 and the Z value is minus 2.0 or greater, the total post-repair PRV/LV is likely to be less than 0.8. Our experience and that of others has indicated that a PRV/LV of 0.8 or less in the operating room is likely to give a late post-repair PRV/LV of 0.7 or less, and in this situation a transannular patch is generally not needed.

The Effect of Transannular Patching

Although the evidence is not conclusive, the data from *Wessel* et al. [5] indicate that pulmonary incompetence induced by transannular patching may be deleterious to late postoperative exercise tolerance, especially when combined with cardiomegaly. Also, in our institution at least, transannular patching is associated with an increased risk of hospital death after complete repair in the first 2 years of life [11].

Between 1972 and 1978, 194 patients underwent correction of tetralogy of Fallot under a protocol of routine primary repair for symptomatic infants (table IV). The mortality for patients without transannular patching was 3.4 versus 14% among patients who required a transannular patch, a highly significant difference. These groups were then compared with a two-stage group which included 158 patients who had undergone previous Blalock-Taussig or Waterston shunts (fig. 4) [11]. In the presence of transannular patching, the risk of primary repair increases markedly at very young ages. Analysis of this data indicates that in our institution a two-stage repair is safer than a primary repair when a transannular patch is needed for patients less than about 24 months of age. When a transannular patch is *not* required, however, two-stage repair is safer than primary repair only when the patient is both very young and very small, less than about 0.35 m^2.

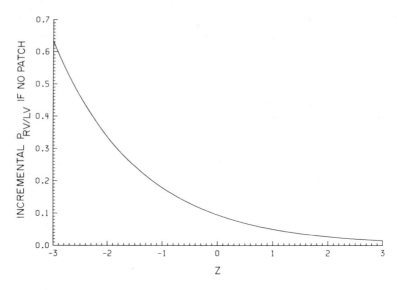

Fig.3. Nomogram representing the incremental $P_{RV/LV}$ if no transannular patch is used, related to Z [from ref. 9].

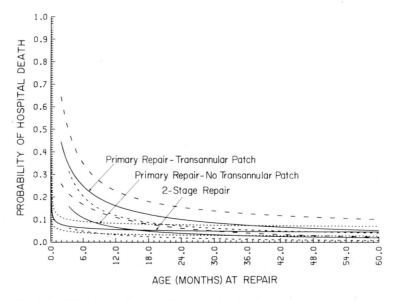

Fig.4. Simplified comparison of the hospital mortality (with 70% confidence limits) of primary repair and that of the two-stage repair, using only age at operation and transannular patch (yes-no) at primary repair [from ref. 11].

Table IV. Classic tetralogy of Fallot. Primary repair without major associated lesions (UAB 1972–1978)

No transannular patch				Transannular patch				Total			
	hospital deaths				hospital deaths				hospital deaths		
n	n	%	70% CL, %	n	n	%	70% CL, %	n	n	%	70% CL, %
117	4	3.4	1.7–6.1	74	10	14	9–19	194	15	7.7	5.7–10.2

CL = Confidence limits; UAB = University of Alabama, Birmingham.

Choice of Palliative Operation

In most reports favoring early primary correction, an important mortality has been ascribed to early palliative shunting for tetralogy of Fallot. *Stephenson* et al. [12] reviewed a number of series of palliative operations for tetralogy, and noted a 40% mortality in the first 3 months of life, 26% in the first 6 months of life, and 22% in the first 12 months of life.

This, however, has not been the experience at the University of Alabama. Certainly if one chooses to perform palliative operations for selected patients with tetralogy of Fallot early in life, it is essential to utilize a procedure which has a very low operative mortality, minimal morbidity, and results in nearly uniform survival until the time of complete correction.

Because of the potential for important kinking of the right pulmonary artery after Waterston anastomosis, and because of the greater tendency to produce congestive heart failure, we routinely perform a classical or modified Blalock-Taussig shunt as the procedure of choice when initial palliation is selected. The overall patency rate is excellent, congestive heart failure is rare, and ligation of the shunt at time of total correction is generally uncomplicated. Analysis of the experience from our institution and from *Arciniegas* et al. [13] in Detroit for classical shunting operations as part of a two-stage repair of tetralogy of Fallot with or without pulmonary atresia indicates that the results from 1967 to 1978 are quite good. 149 patients underwent initial shunting procedures for symptomatic tetralogy in the first 2 years of life with 6 deaths for an operative mortality of 4%. The choice of shunt between Blalock and Waterston had no effect on hospital mortality, nor did the presence or absence of pulmonary atresia. Note that no patients surviving the initial postoperative period died before the age of 3 years.

The results of classical Blalock-Taussig shunts in the first 1–4 weeks of life, however, have not been totally satisfactory. The patency rate is not uniformly good, there is a rather high incidence of distortion of the pulmonary artery by a rather short subclavian segment, and the quality and size of the subclavian artery are variable when used in the first 1–4 weeks of life.

We believe that the palliative operation of choise for tetralogy of Fallot in the first month of life is a modified Blalock-Taussig shunt using Gore-Tex from the undivided subclavian artery to the pulmonary artery. *Donahoo* et al. [14] at Johns Hopkins University in 1980 reported the use of poly-tetrafluorethylene (Gore-Tex) shunts for palliative shunting in the first month of life. Their series included 16 patients under 1 month of age with various forms of cyanotic congenital heart disease. They utilized the subclavian or innominate artery or the descending aorta for the proximal anastomosis and the right or left pulmonary artery for the distal anastomosis. They advocated α-adrenergic support if the systolic pressure was less than 90 mm Hg, routinely administered heparin in a dose of 1 mg/kg at the time of shunt construction, and used a 4-mm Gore-Tex shunt in the first month of life.

Of these 16 patients, there were 2 hospital deaths, both of whom had patent shunts, and follow-up ranging from 4 months to 3.5 years revealed only one late shunt occlusion. Subsequent to this report, anecdotal evidence from a number of surgeons has suggested that a 5- or 6-mm Gore-Tex shunt is probably the optimal size in patients in the first month of life.

The current results of palliative shunting in the first 2 years of life at our institution since 1978 are indicated in table V. We believe that this very low mortality is consistent with our goals of avoiding deaths before the patient undergoes complete correction.

Transatrial versus Transventricular Repair

The matter of transatrial versus transventricular repair for tetralogy of Fallot remains controversial. *Edmunds* et al. [15] at the University of Pennsylvania published a favorable experience with transatrial repair of tetralogy in 1976. We have been rather late to utilize the transatrial approach, but currently have a small ongoing experience with transatrial repair of tetralogy, and we believe that it will be most useful in selected patients with isolated infundibular stenosis who will not require a transannular patch.

Optimal Timing for Elective Repair

Although the precise optimal timing for elective repair of tetralogy is unknown, late follow-up studies suggest that repair should probably not be

Table V. Shunts for classical tetralogy of Fallot ($<$ 2 years) (UAB, 1978–1981)

n	Hospital deaths		
	n	%	70% CL, %
15	0	0	0–12

Table VI. Management program for tetralogy of Fallot

1	Patient $>$ 2 years of age: primary repair
2	Symptomatic patient $<$ 2 years of age:

If *no transannular patch* needed, primary repair at any age unless patient is both very young and very small ($<$ 0.35 m²)

If *transannular patch* needed, Blalock-Taussig shunt (Gortex in first month of life) followed by complete repair at age 2–4 years

delayed past about 5 years of age, and we currently recommend elective repair at about 2–4 years of age.

Patient Management Program for Tetralogy of Fallot

In selecting a patient management program for the treatment of patients with the tetralogy of Fallot, it is important to again recall the lessons that we have learned from the long-term follow-up studies. If our patients survive the period up to and shortly after complete repair, they are very likely to have an excellent long-term result. With this in mind, the current recommended management program at our institution for patients with symptomatic tetralogy of Fallot is indicated in table VI. If the patient is greater than 2 years of age, primary complete repair is recommended. If the patient is less than 2 years of age, and our measurements from the angiogram indicate that a transannular patch will not be necessary, then again primary repair is recommended essentially at any age, unless the patient is both extremely young and very small (less than about 0.35 m²). If our measurements, however, indicate that a transannular patch will be needed in the first 2 years of life, our data indicate that the combined mortality of the palliative operation plus the later complete repair will be less than that of a primary repair. In this situation we would recommend initial palliative shunting with a classical Blalock-Taussig shunt, or in a patient less than about 1 month of age a Gore-Tex shunt, followed by a complete repair at about 2–4 years of age.

References

1   Bertranou, E.G.; Blackstone, E.H.; Haxelrig, J.B.; Turner, M.E., Jr.; Kirklin, J.W.: Life expectancy without surgery in the tetralogy of Fallot. Am.J.Cardiol.*42:* 458 (1978).

2   Fuster, V.; McGoon, D.C.; Kennedy, M.A.; Ritter, D.G.; Kirklin, J.W.: Long-term evaluation (12–22 years) of open heart surgery for tetralogy of Fallot. Am.J. Cardiol.*46:* 635 (1980).

3   Katz, N.M.; Blackstone, E.H.; Kirklin, J.W.; Pacifico, A.D.; Bargeron, L.M., Jr.: Survival and symptoms late after repair of tetralogy of Fallot. Circulation (in press).

4   Rocchini, A.P.; Rosenthal, A.; Freed, M.; Castaneda, A.R.; Nadas, A.S.: Chronic congestive heart failure after repair of tetralogy of Fallot. Circulation *56:* 305 (1977).

5   Wessel, H.U.; Cunningham, W.J.; Paul, M.H.; Bastanier, C.K.; Muster, A.J.; Idriss, F.S.: Exercise performance in tetralogy of Fallot after intracardiac repair. J.thorac.cardiovasc.Surg.*80:* 582 (1980).

6   Lillehei, C.W.; Cohen, M.; Warden, H.E.; Varco, R.L.: The direct vision intra-cardiac correction of congenital anomalies by controlled cross circulation. Surgery, St Louis *38:* 11 (1955).

7   Barratt-Boyes, B.G.; Neutze, J.M.: Primary repair of tetralogy of Fallot in infancy using profound hypothermia with circulatory arrest and limited cardiopulmonary bypass: a comparison with conventional two stage management. Ann.Surg.*178:* 406 (1973).

8   Rowlatt, U.F.; Rimoldi, H.J.A.; Lev, H.: The quantitative anatomy of the normal child's heart. Pediat. Clins N.Am.*10:* 499 (1963).

9   Blackstone, E.H.; Kirklin, J.W.; Bertranou, E.G.; Labrosse, C.J.; Soto, B.; Bargeron, L.M., Jr.: Preoperative prediction from cineangiograms of postrepair right ventricular pressure in tetralogy of Fallot. J.thorac.cardiovasc.Surg.*78:* 542 (1979).

10 Blackstone, E.H.; Kirklin, J.W.; Pacifico, A.D.: Decision-making in the repair of tetralogy of Fallot based on intraoperative measurements of the pulmonary arterial outflow tract. J.thorac.cardiovasc.Surg.*77:* 526 (1979).

11 Kirklin, J.W.; Blackstone, E.H.; Pacifico, A.D.; Brown, R.N.; Bargeron, L.M., Jr.: Routine primary repair vs two-stage repair of tetralogy of Fallot. Circulation *60:* 373 (1979).

12 Stephenson, L.W.; Friedman, S.; Edmunds, L.H., Jr.: Staged surgical management of tetralogy of Fallot in infants. Circulation *58:* 837 (1978).

13 Arciniegas, E.; Blackstone, E.H.; Pacifico, A.D.; Kirklin, J.W.: Classic shunting operations as part of two-stage repair for tetralogy of Fallot. Ann.thor.Surg.*27:* 514 (1979).

14 Donahoo, J.S.; Garner, T.J.; Zahkak, S.; Langforkidd, B.S.: Systemic-pulmonary artery shunt in neonates and infants using microporous expanded polytetrafluoroehylene: immediate and late results. Ann.thorac.Surg. *30:* 146 (1980).
15 Edmunds, L.H.; Saxena, N.C.; Friedman, S.; Rashkind, W.J.; Dodd, P.F.: Transatrial resection of the obstructed right ventricular infundibulum. Circulation *54:* 117 (1976).
16 Pacifico, A.D.; Kirklin, J.W.; Blackstone, E.H.: Surgical management of pulmonary stenosis in tetralogy of Fallot. J.thor.cardiovasc.Surg. *74:* 382 (1977).

James K. Kirklin, MD, Department of Surgery, Division of Cardiovascular and Thoracic Surgery, University of Alabama in Birmingham, University Station, Birmingham, AL 35233 (USA)

Mod. Probl. Paediat., vol. 22, pp. 152–156 (Karger, Basel 1983)

Correction of Tetralogy of Fallot by Combined Transatrial and Pulmonary Approach

J. P. Binet[a], *L. Patane*[b], *R. Nottin*[a]

[a] Hôpital Marie-Lannelongue, Le Plessis-Robinson, Paris, France;
[b] Divisione di Cardiochirurgia, Ospedale Vittorio Emanuele II, Catania, Italia

Introduction

Right ventricular heart failure is one of the major problems after complete correction of the tetralogy of Fallot (TF). In order to minimize aggression to the right ventricle, repair was carried out through the right atrium and the pulmonary artery, thus avoiding right ventriculotomy. 136 consecutive cases of TF have been operated upon from 1979 to 1981 without opening the right ventricle and we think this is a suitable technique for any anatomic configuration of TF provided the infant is at least 6 months old (fig. 1). Patient age ranged from 7 months to 28 years. 43 patients were under 2 years old at the time of operation.

Operative Technique

Through a median sternotomy, cardiopulmonary bypass is established. The aorta is cross-clamped and myocardial and body protection is provided by profound hypothermia, cardioplegic (Bretschneider) and topical cooling. Myocardial temperature is monitored and the left ventricle is vented through the apex.

During the infusion of the cardioplegic solution, we perform a large, high, horizontal atriotomy, through which the atrial and ventricular septal defects (ASD and VSD) are closed and low right ventricle hypertrophy is resected. The VSD is closed with a Teflon patch secured with interrupted mattress sutures over Teflon pladgets; the stitches are put on the edge of the VSD or on the right aspect of the ventricular septum. The resection of the low

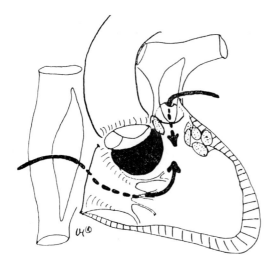

Fig. 1. Tetralogy of Fallot. Schematic representation of the right ventricle. Ventricular septal defect in subaortic position can be closed through the tricuspid orifice. Infundibular hypertrophy may be resected via the tricuspid orifice or the pulmonary trunk after correction of pulmonary valvular stenosis.

infundibular hypertrophy is achieved using a special dissector. Each muscular bundle is cut individually. After incision of the pulmonary trunk, measurements are made of the trunk, both pulmonary arteries and the pulmonary annulus.

At this stage there are two possibilities: (1) The annulus is not restrictive: we resect the superior infundibular hypertrophy through the pulmonary valve. (2) The annulus is restrictive according to the tables of Kirklin and Pacifico: we incise the annulus and a small part of infundibulum (3–4 mm).

Finally, when necessary, the pulmonary artery and the branches are enlarged with a pericardial patch.

Results

We used this technique in 136 consecutive cases of TF. The patients are separated in to two groups, according to whether or not the pulmonary annulus was divided.

Table I. Conservation of the pulmonary annulus (not opened), 52/136 cases (0 = death)

	Cases
Total correction through right atrium *only*	2
Total correction through right atrium and longitudinal arteriotomy	32
Total correction through right atrium and angioplastic enlargement	
of pulmonary artery	18
Main pulmonary artery	13
Main pulmonary artery and left pulmonary artery	5
Bifurcation	0

Table II. Opening of the pulmonary annulus, 84/136 cases (9 deaths)

	Cases
Valvulotomy and pulmonary infundibulotomy (3–4 mm)	
Pulmonary reconstruction (pericardium, *never* Dacron)	
Main pulmonary artery	19
Main pulmonary artery and left pulmonary artery	45
Bifurcation	20
With transection of the aorta	5
Cause of the death (9)	
Sepsis	
Low cardiac output (insufficient protection of the myocardium, before 1980)	
Sudden death	

Group I. 52 patients (38 %) did not have the annulus divided (table I). Among these, the correction was performed in 2 patients through atrial incision alone. In 50 the correction was carried out through both atrial and pulmonary incisions. 18 of these patients required enlargement of the pulmonary artery (13 main pulmonary artery, 5 main pulmonary artery and left pulmonary artery). There has been no mortality among this patient group.

Group II. 84 patients (62 %) required division of the pulmonary annulus (table II). The infundibulum and the pulmonary artery were enlarged with a pericardial patch (19 main pulmonary artery, 45 main pulmonary artery and left pulmonary artery, 20 pulmonary bifurcation with temporary division of the aorta in 5 cases). We had 9 deaths in this group (5 low cardiac output, 3 sepsis, 1 sudden death).

Table III. 'Complicated' Fallot with associated anomalies, 15 cases (1 death)

	Cases
Left obstructive cardiomyopathy	1
Left ventricular OD fistula	1
Multiple ventricular septal defects	2
Pulmonary valvular agenesis	1
Left coronary artery arising from the right coronary artery	9
WPW	1

Table IV. Right ventricular pressure

After bypass
  60–70 % of aortic pressure

After closure of the sternotomy
  Always < 50 % of aortic pressure

Postoperative catheterization (32 cases)
  30 % of aortic pressure – whatever anatomic type

Using the same technique, we have treated 15 cases of TF with associated pathology. There was 1 death in this group: a case with multiple VSD (table III).

In 9 patients an anomalous left coronary artery passed in front of the right ventricular infundibulum. We had no trouble in respecting this artery. Postoperative pressure measurements are shown in table IV.

Discussion

The procedure we describe above is relatively simple to perform. The non-hemorrhagic part of the operation (ASD and VSD closure, resection of the low infundibular hypertrophy) can be carried out during cooling. The hemorrhagic part can be performed when profound hypothermia is achieved and pump flow can be reduced. This technique has been successfully employed in every kind of anatomic configuration of TF, with and without associated anomalies. We believe there is no danger of damage to the atrioventricular conduction system, as we have not encountered any complete atrioventricular block. In 2 cases with bifascicular block a pacemaker was implanted. Postoperative intracardiac and pulmonary pressures were satisfactory when measured. Postoperative recovery was shorter and required a briefer period of assisted ventilation. We employed the transatrial and transpulmonary route in order to protect the right ventricle. More follow up and a comparative study is needed to conclude whether or not this goal is reached. The preliminary results of postperative catheterization and isotopic studies appear to be better than in patients operated via right ventriculotomy.

J.P. Binet, Chief in Cardiovascular Surgery, Hôpital Marie-Lannelongue, 133, Avenue de la Résistance, F-92350 Le Plessis-Robinson (France)

Mod. Probl. Paediat., vol. 22, pp. 157–161 (Karger, Basel 1983)

The Utility of a Monocusp Patch to Relieve the Right Ventricular Outflow Tract Obstruction in Tetralogy of Fallot Corrected in Infancy

Gian Piero Piccoli

Royal Liverpool Children's Hospital, Liverpool, England

At the Royal Liverpool Children's Hospital, between February 1969 and March 1980, 235 patients, ranging in age from 5 months to 18 years (mean $\pm$ 5.7 years), underwent total repair of tetralogy of Fallot. There were 18 hospital deaths (early mortality rate = 7.6%).

The relation between the age at operation and the early mortality was significant in those who underwent operation prior to 1977 (fig. 1). Of the 23 patients less than 2 years of age in the period 1969–1976, 6 (26%) died in the hospital, compared with 8 early deaths (5%) among 152 cases in the older age group ($p < 0.001$). However, since 1977, there have been no deaths in 17 consecutive infants submitted to primary repair. During the first period of this experience, a conservative policy to relieve the right ventricular outflow tract (RVOT) obstruction was followed; subsequently, a more aggressive policy was adopted (table I). Overall, the early mortality was significantly higher when a transannular approach was used (9 out of 41 cases, 22%) than when the pulmonary valve annulus was preserved (9 out of 194 cases, 4.5%) ($p < 0.0001$) (table I). However, since 1977, the use of a transannular gusset has been associated with a lower mortality rate (2 out of 18 cases, 11%) when compared with the previous period (4 out of 15 cases, 26%). Furthermore, the use of a transannular patch in cases less than 2 years has not been associated with a higher hospital mortality (fig. 2).

Among the 23 infants who underwent total repair before 1977, transannular approach was not performed while, among the 17 patients under 2 years of age who underwent intracardiac repair during the last 4 years, a

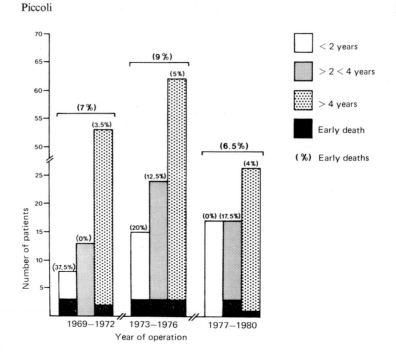

Fig.1. Years of operation related to age of patients at operation.

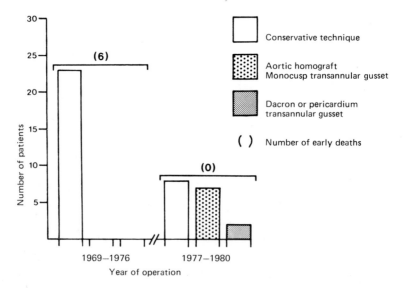

Fig.2. Surgical relief of right ventricular outflow tract obstruction in patients less than 2 years of age.

Table I. Surgical relief of right ventricular outflow tract obstruction

	Patients during the period 1968–1976			Patients during the period 1977–1980			Total	
	number	%	early deaths	number	%	early deaths	number	early deaths
Infundibulectomy	65	37	5	12	20		77	5
Infundibulectomy and infundibular gusset	5	3	1				5	1
Infundibulectomy and pulmonary valvotomy	86	49	3	26	43.5		112	3
Dacron or pericardium transannular gusset	11	6	2	6	10	1	17	3
Aortic homograft monoscup trans- annular gusset	4	2.5	2	12	20	1	16	3
Inlayed aortic homograft conduit	4	2.5	1	4	6.5	2	8	3

transannular approach was performed in 9 (fig. 2). In 7 of these infants, an aortic monocusp gusset was used to relieve the RVOT obstruction. The monocusp patch is obtained from a fresh, antibiotic preserved, homograft conduit. This is longitudinally opened and a piece of aortic wall, the under-lying mitral valve with the non-coronary aortic cusp are then resected (fig. 3, 4).

The 13 survivors in whom an aortic homograft monocusp patch was utilized, have been regularly reviewed in our out-patient clinic with a mean follow-up of ± 22 months. Its use was never found associated with late symptoms and all cases were leading a normal life, in a accordance with their age, although a faint diastolic murmur was present in 2 instances. Cardiac catheterization was performed in 4 of them, as part of a routine post-operative haemodynamic evaluation. The overall contractility of the right ventricle appeared normal, without residual gradient at RVOT level. With-drawal tracings revealed almost a normal diastolic pressure in the pulmonary artery with a gradient of more than 8 mm Hg between the mid-diastolic

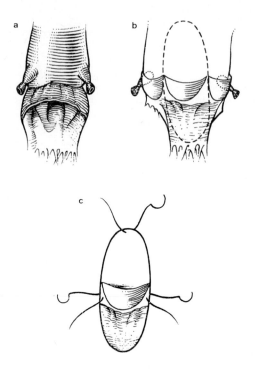

Fig.3. Method of preparation of the aortic homograft monocusp patch. A fresh, antibiotic preserved, aortic homograft *(a)* is longitudinally opened *(b).* A piece of aortic wall and the underlying mitral valve with the non-coronary aortic valve cusp are then resected *(c).*

pressures of the main pulmonary artery and of the right ventricle. Injecting the contrast medium into the main pulmonary artery, in all 4 patients there was only a minimal regurgitant stream opacifying the RVOT (probably caused by the catheter) which was cleared out in every case in one or two cycles from the end of the injection. It may be concluded that aortic homograft monocusp gusset allows a more aggressive policy in the surgical

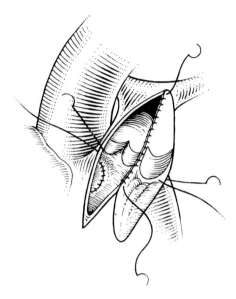

Fig.4. Right ventricular outflow tract reconstruction using a transannular aortic monocusp gusset.

treatment of TF, relieving satisfactorily the obstruction and preventing the early free pulmonary incompetence. Late diastolic murmur could be due to the imperfect alignment of the monocusp with the patient's own cusps, although late shrinkage of the monocusp tissue cannot be excluded.

In view of these results, the suggested policy for patients with TF in our unit is as follows: (1) palliative procedures in infants under 6 months of age and in cases with diminutive pulmonary arteries; (2) early total repair in infants older than 6 months and with favourable anatomy; (3) an aortic monocusp homograft is a preferable choice whenever a transannular approach is required.

Gian Piero Piccoli, MD, Ospedale Specializzato Regionale, "G.M.Lancisi", Via Baccarani 6, I–60100 Ancona (Italy)

Mod. Probl. Paediat., vol. 22, pp. 162–166 (Karger, Basel 1983)

Pulmonary Atresia with Intact Ventricular Septum

George A. Trusler[a], *Robert M. Freedom*[b]

[a] Department of Surgery, University of Toronto School of Medicine, and Division of Cardiovascular Surgery, The Hospital for Sick Children, Toronto;
[b] Department of Pediatrics and Pathology, University of Toronto School of Medicine, and The Hospital for Sick Children, Toronto, Ontario, Canada

In early years, some form of pulmonary valvotomy or a systemic pulmonary shunt was the basic palliation for pulmonary atresia with intact ventricular septum. Results were poor with only 2 long-term survivors in our series. Since 1968, we employed a broader approach which included: (1) balloon atrial septostomy at cardiac catheterization, followed by (2) a systemic pulmonary artery shunt, usually a Pott's anastomosis, and, at the same time, (3) a transarterial pulmonary valvotomy. If the shunt was functioning well, the patent ductus arteriosus was ligated, particularly if it was large. Our experience with this broader scheme of management was reported in 1978, and included 37 patients with some indication of the longer-term results and problems [5]. Since 1978, another 14 infants have been operated on, making a total of 51 patients in this recent group.

Clinical Material

From 1968 to 1980, 56 patients with pulmonary atresia and intact ventricular septum were operated on at the Hospital for Sick Children, Toronto. There were 25 males and 31 females. 54 were neonates of whom 50 were less than 1 week old at operation. By angiocardiography, 51 had a small to diminutive right ventricle and were managed as described. Those with even a pinhole opening in the pulmonary valve at operation or autopsy were not included in this series. 5 infants had a small normal-to-large right ventricle and all had severe tricuspid incompetence. In this small group, pulmonary valvotomy was often not sufficient and many need reconstruction of the right ventricular outflow tract, as well as the tricuspid valve. In fact, some need tricuspid valve replacement. 2 of these 5 children survived, but only because they had better than average tricuspid valves.

All but 1 of the 51 infants with small right ventricle had balloon atrial septostomy at cardiac catheterization. At operation, 49 had systemic pulmonary artery anastomoses: 34 Pott's, 4 left Blalock-Taussig, 1 right Blalock-Taussig, 3 Waterston and 7 central aortopulmonary anastomoses (table I). 27 had a patent ductus arteriosus ligation and 32 had a transarterial pulmonary valvotomy at the same operation. 2 infants with unusually mild infundibular stenosis had only a transventricular pulmonary valvotomy.

A second palliative procedure was performed on 12 children, including 8 shunts and 1 shunt revision. 6 of the 9 children who had a second shunt, also had a transventricular pulmonary valvotomy at the same operation and 3 other children had a pulmonary valvotomy without a shunt. There were 3 deaths in these 12 cases. It appeared that the mortality with the original shunt procedure and pulmonary valvotomy plus the secondary palliative procedure could be effective. In fact, it appeared that the palliative approach would keep three quarters of the children alive.

Change to a More Aggressive Philosophy

With increasing experience, and with the development of the Fontan operation, it became apparent that patients with pulmonary atresia and intact ventricular septum should be repaired by reconstruction of the right ventricular outflow tract if the right ventricle grows to an adequate size. If the right ventricle does not grow, the long-term plan should be atrial pulmonary diversion, in other words, some form of Fontan procedure.

It had been our hope that a shunt plus pulmonary valvotomy, by creating pulmonary incompetence, would stimulate an increase in right ventricular volume. However, *Patel* et al. [4] reviewed 18 of our patients who had preoperative and postoperative right ventricular angiocardiograms to estimate the change in right ventricular volume. 10 showed some increase in right ventricular size, but only 5 of the 10 had a right ventricle that was normal or larger than normal in size. When the change in right ventricular volume was correlated with the anatomic lesion, it appeared that the greatest stimulus to growth was tricuspid incompetence. However, most of our cases did not have adequate relief of the right ventricular obstruction, and it is possible that a more effective pulmonary valvotomy would have stimulated better right ventricular growth.

Table I. Pulmonary atresia, small right ventricle, 1968–1980

Primary operation		Patent ductus arteriosus ligation	Pulmonary valvotomy	Survived
Potts	34	25	24	26
Central aortopulmonary anastomosis	7	2	6	6
Left Blalock-Taussig	4		2	1
Right Blalock-Taussig	1			1
Waterston	3			2
Pulmonary valvotomy	2			2
	51			38 (75%)

1 death 10 months later, after cardiac catheterization – excessive shunt.

Since adequate right ventricular growth was obtained by only a few patients, it seemed that some type of Fontan repair should be considered as the ultimate operation for most of these children. Adequate pulmonary artery size is one of the major needs for an adequate Fontan repair. While our early experience with the Pott's shunt was excellent with low mortality and good long-term palliation, we encountered a substantial incidence of late pulmonary artery stenosis of a degree of severity which made a Fontan operation difficult or impossible. As a result of this reevaluation in 1978, we changed from the Pott's shunt to other shunts. In particular we have used central shunts, or more recently the Goretex shunts between the subclavian artery and pulmonary artery described by *de Leval* et al. [1]. Both of those shunts are more difficult and less sure than the Pott's but associated with fewer late problems.

Another major necessity for a Fontan operation is good left ventricular function. In order to preserve this, the right ventricle must be decompressed. In our series, 18 children had right ventricular pressure measured at a second cardiac catheterization. Some of these were before and some after a second palliative procedure. The right ventricular pressure was close to normal in 2 children and moderately elevated in another 2. In the other 14 children, there was elevation to systemic or suprasystemic levels. With good angio-cardiography, the exact site of the lesion could be identified and was usually infundibular, although sometimes it was valvular and infundibular. The double catheter technique with one catheter in the right ventricle and one in the pulmonary artery was sometimes useful in clarifying the cause of obstruction in difficult cases [3].

Often the angiogram would reveal myocardial sinusoids connecting the lumen of the right ventricle with the coronary artery system. This sinister connection allowed cyanotic blood from the right ventricle to perfuse the myocardium and cause myocardial fibrosis. These sinusoidal connections are sometimes seen soon after birth and likely they develop as a result of high right ventricular pressure. Thus, they constitute an extra indication for early repair of right ventricular outflow tract obstruction in this condition. Unfortunately, flow through the sinusoids may reverse after the right ventricular pressure is reduced, allowing a steal or reversal of blood flow from the coronary arteries into the right ventricle.

Reconstruction of the Right Ventricular Outflow Tract

With the more aggressive philosophy, and with the realization that any long-term future for these patients involves a right ventricular outflow tract reconstruction, either to stimulate growth of the right ventricle, or merely to decompress it, so that atrial pulmonary diversion could be done in the future, we embarked on a program similar to that advocated by *Dobell and Grignon* [2] in which a right ventricular outflow tract reconstruction was carried out as early as 6 months of age.

The right ventricular ouflow tract was reconstructed in 18 patients (table II). In 6 patients, there had been some evidence of right ventricular growth which allowed us to approach the anatomic problem as if doing a partial or complete repair. In these cases, we not only reconstructed the outflow tract, but we partially or completely repaired the shunt and/or the atrial septal defect. 3 of the 6 patients survived, 2 with a degree of temporary right heart failure. 1 of the children who died had a right atrial to right ventricular conduit, because the tricuspid valve was very small.

In another 6 patients, there had been little growth of the right ventricle and the right ventricular pressure was at or above systemic levels. We attempted to bring this pressure down to normal levels by patching the right ventricular outflow tract. All 6 children died in myocardial failure at, or soon after, the operation.

In 6 other children, the right ventricular outflow tract was reconstructed using a valve and a patch. These patients were similar to the last 6, in that they all had high right ventricular pressures. A valve was inserted to prevent

Table II. Right ventricular outflow tract reconstruction

Operation	Number	Survived
Partial or complete repair	5	3
Atriopulmonary diversion	1	0
Right ventricular outflow tract patch	6	0
Right ventricular outflow tract patch and valve	6	3
	18	6 (33%)

back flow across the outflow tract. Reverse flow was a concern, either because the aortopulmonary shunt was large or centrally placed, or because there was an incompetent tricuspid valve. There were 3 early survivors following this operation. 1 died at a second operation to narrow an excessive shunt. It is difficult to compare this group of 6 children with the previous group of 6 children. While superficial comparison suggests that these children are better with insertion of a valve, the difference is really more involved with many factors to be considered. The high mortality with right ventricular outflow tract reconstruction demands different and possibly earlier operations.

References

1   deLeval, M.R.; McKay, R.; Jones, M.; Stark, H.; Macartney, F.J.: Modified Blalock-Taussig shunt. J.thorac.cardiovasc.Surg.*81:* 112 (1981).
2   Dobell, A.R.C.; Grignon, A.: Early and late results in pulmonary atresia. Ann. thor.Surg.*24:* 264 (1977).
3   Freedom, R.M.; White, R.I., Jr.; Ho, C.S.; Gingell, R.L.; Hawker, R.E.; Rowe, R.D.: Evaluation of patients with pulmonary atresia and intact ventricular septum by double catheter technique. Am.J.Cardiol.*33:* 892 (1974).
4   Patel, R.G.; Freedom, R.M.; Moes, C.A.F.; Bloom, K.R.; Olley, P.M.; Williams, W.G.; Trusler, G.A.; Rowe, R.D.: Right ventricular volume determinations in 18 patients with pulmonary atresia and intact ventricular septum. Analysis of factors influencing right ventricular growth. Circulation *61:* 428 (1980).
5   Trusler, G.A.; Freedom, R.M.; Patel, R.; Williams, W.G.: Surgical management of pulmonary atresia with intact ventricular septum. In: Godman and Marquis (eds.) Paediatric cardiology – heart disease in the newborn, vol.2, chap.23, p.305 (Churchill Livingstone, Edinburgh 1979).

George A.Trusler, MD, Associate Professor of Surgery, University of Toronto School of Medicine, Head, Division of Cardiovascular Surgery, The Hospital for Sick Children, Toronto, Ont. (Canada)

Mod. Probl. Paediat., vol. 22, pp. 167–185 (Karger, Basel 1983)

Surgical Treatment of Pulmonary Atresia with Right Ventricular Hypoplasia and Intact Septum

Peter B. Mansfield, Dale G. Hall, Edward A. Rittenhouse, Lester R. Sauvage, Stanley J. Stamm, S. Paul Herndon

Children's Orthopedic Hospital and Medical Center, Seattle, Wash., USA

Introduction

The outlook for infants born with pulmonary atresia with right ventricular (RV) hypoplasia and an intact ventricular septum is poor [1–13]. Dependent on a patent ductus for survival, these infants are usually profoundly hypoxic at birth. Cardiac arrest is frequently seen during diagnostic efforts and initial palliative surgery. For those who survive, late deaths are frequent [1, 2, 4, 7, 9, 12, 13], and those patients who survive subsequent procedures do not look forward to a normal existence [3, 19]. Because of this bleak outlook for these infants, we have developed a sequential surgical approach aimed toward a complete anatomic and physiologic repair of this defect, without the use of artificial materials or devices. This report reviews our experience initiated in 1973 and describes the surgical sequence of the first 7 patients who survived to undergo complete surgical correction.

Clinical Data

23 critically ill hypoxic infants were admitted to Children's Orthopedic Hospital and Medical Center (COHMC) between June 1973 and June 1978 and at emergency catheterization were shown to have pulmonary atresia or pinhole critical pulmonary stenosis. In addition several had hypoplastic or small RV. 7 of these patients with hypoplastic or small, thick-walled RV and either pulmonary atresia (5) or critical pulmonary stenosis (2) have completed a sequence of surgical procedures leading to RV enlargement, the

Table I. Initial clinical presentation

Case No.	Age at admission, days	Arrest	Cyanosis	CHF	Murmurs	EKG	Chest X-Ray	
							pulmonary vascularity	right atrial size
1	1	× 1	++	no	PDA TI	LVH	↓	↑↑
2	4	no	+++	no	?TI	RAH LVH	↓	↑↑
3	3	× 2	+++	yes	no heart sounds	RAH LVH	↓ ↓	↑↑
4	1	no	+	no	PDA	RVH	normal	↑
5	5	no	++	no	PDA TI	RAH RVH	normal	↑↑
6	1	no	+	no	PDA ?TI	RAH RVH	normal	↑
7	23	no	+	no	PDA TI	LVH	normal	↑

CHF = congestive heart failure;
LVH = left ventricular hypoplasia; RVH = right ventricular hypoplasia;
RAH = right atrial hypoplasia;
PDA = patent ductus arteriosus;
TI = tricuspid insufficiency.

creation of a functional pulmonary valve and total anatomic repair of their defect. These 7 comprise the group studied in this paper.

The clinical presentation of these infants is shown in table I. All were noted to be cyanotic within 24 h of birth. 2 of the 7 had at least one cardiac arrest prior to initiation of their shunt surgery. At the initial cardiac catheterization an atrial balloon septostomy was performed whenever there was evidence of a restrictive atrial septal defect (ASD) (fig. 1).

Surgical Considerations

Initial Treatment

The surgical sequence used in these patients is shown in table II. No oxygen was administrated in the hospital until a patent aortopulmonary shunt was functioning. Cardiac catheterization was performed immediately

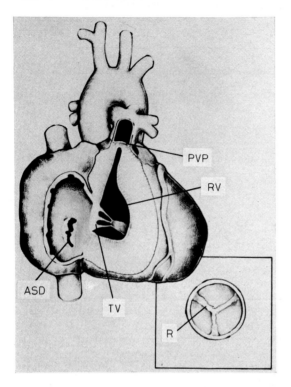

Fig. 1. The anatomy of a typical pulmonary atresia with a hypoplastic or small right ventricle and an intact septum is shown in a cut-away section. A balloon atrial septostomy (ASD) has already been performed. Note the small right ventricular chamber (RV), thick right ventricular wall, and small but adequate tricuspid valve (TV). There are no sinuses of Valsalva seen at the pulmonary valve plate (PVP). The insert shows a view of the valve plate as seen from the main pulmonary artery. Note the ridges (R) which conform to typical distribution of commissures. As in the majority of cases of pulmonary atresia with an intact ventricular septum the main pulmonary artery is of near normal size.

and the infants were taken directly to surgery following the rapid diagnostic procedure. Prostaglandin E_1 was used on the last 2 patients in this group when it first became available to us.

The goal of the initial hospitalization was to increase pulmonary blood flow and to decompress the RV in a manner which would also lead to mild pulmonary insufficiency. Since aortic insufficiency leads to enlargement of the left ventricle (LV) in other clinical situations, it was hoped the same would be obtained for the hypoplastic or small RV in these infants.

Table II. Surgical sequence for providing pulmonary blood flow and subsequent right ventricular enlargement

Treatment	Age	Concept
No ↑ FIO₂ prostaglandin E₁ infusion	newborn	Keep ductus patent until shunt functioning
Catheterization; ? balloon atrial septostomy	newborn	diagnosis: ASD creation if restrictive
Aortopulmonary shunt	newborn	↑ pulmonary blood flow, PO₂ (prefer Blalock)
Core decompression	< 1 month	1 create mild PI 2 decompress RV (↓ RVEDP) 3 ↑ MPA blood flow 4 ↓ TR 5 enlarge RV with time 6 create functional pulmonary valve
Total anatomic repair	2–3 years	use enlarged RV and formed pulmonary valve to complete repair

ASD = Atrial septal defect;   PI = pulmonary insufficiency;   RVEDP = right ventricular end-diastolic pressure;   TR = tricuspid regurgitation.

Blind transventricular pulmonary valvotomy has not been uniformly successful in opening the outflow tract and/or valve plate in the past, and rarely creates pulmonary insufficiency [1, 2, 7, 19]. We devised a closed heart technique (core decompression) to core out and remove a central portion of the pulmonary valve plate under direct vision without compromising cardiac output. In order to be sure there is adequate pulmonary blood flow during the core decompression and the first few months afterwards, an aortopulmonary shunt is done first.

Aortopulmonary Shunt

We initially used a median sternotomy approach to create a Waterston shunt and perform core decompression of the pulmonary valve plate immediately thereafter. The first 3 patients were done in this way. Although they all survived and have all undergone subsequent successful total repair, we have changed our initial approach to a right thoracotomy for several reasons: (1) It was difficult to create a precisely sized Waterston shunt via a median sternotomy without some kinking of the right pulmonary artery as seen later at subsequent catheterization and at the time of total repair.

(2) The manipulation of the aorta and proximal right pulmonary artery frequently compromised the ductus blood flow and led to ischemic cardiac slowing or arrest during creation of the shunt. (Less a problem since prostaglandin is available.) (3) Clamping of the distal main pulmonary artery (MPA) during core decompression led to decreased shunt flow in 2 patients. When the clamp was moved to permit good shunt flow, the space to work within the MPA was reduced. (4) We have used Blalock shunts in many infants with other types of cyanotic heart disease with excellent results. These shunts provide satisfactory pulmonary flow for about 3 years in our experience, quite long enough to provide adequate pulmonary blood flow for the first few critical months, when the RV stroke volume is increasing. (5) If the subclavian vascular anatomy is inadequate to create a Blalock shunt, a more precise Waterston shunt can be done via the retrocaval route through a right thoracotomy as was done in case 5 whose shunt was approached through the right chest. The Waterston or Blalock shunts are performed in the classic manner.

Core Decompression – Timing and Technique

We feel that RV core decompression should be done soon after the aorto-pulmonary shunt is functioning, the pulmonary vascular resistance has diminished (good systolic and *diastolic* shunt murmur), and the infant is in positive nitrogen balance. This usually takes 1–4 weeks. Cardiac catheterization is done if needed to demonstrate adequate size of the MPA if this is not already known. In our experience almost all patients with pulmonary atresia and an intact ventricular septum have adequate sized MPA.

During the procedure arterial monitoring is used to be sure manipulations are not compromising cardiac output. We keep the arterial pH above 7.4 and avoid base deficits at all times. A xylocaine drip at 20–40 μg/kg/min is maintained to avoid fibrillation from the very thickened RV wall. Calcium is not given because it has produced ventricular fibrillation in at least 2 of these patients with thick-walled RV. An anesthetic technique is used which avoids systemic peripheral vasodilatation, since coupled with a rapid run-off into the lungs via the aortopulmonary shunt, severe intractable hypotension may occur. Intravascular blood volume is kept full.

The surgical technique of core decompression is shown in figures 2–4. The heart is approached via a median sternotomy. The pericardium is opened vertically toward the left side of the mediastinum with the idea of closing it over the ventricle after decompression. This makes the sternotomy for subsequent total repair less hazardous. Mobilization of the MPA may

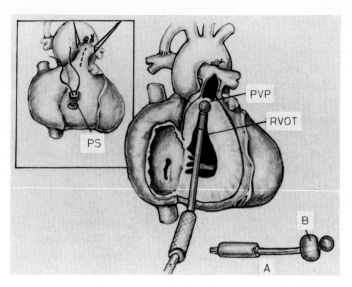

Fig.2. The technique of core decompression of the right ventricular outflow tract is shown. A purse string (PS) is placed near the AV groove on the right ventricle.The purse string must be near the AV groove to successfully enter the right ventricular chamber. After testing for a pin hole leak in the valve plate (see text) the main pulmonary artery is opened and the valve plate visualized. A running closing suture is pre-placed and retracted out of the way. A balloon backed (B) ball tip device (A) is advanced through the purse string into the right ventricular chamber. It is further advanced into the outflow tract of the right ventricle (RVOT) so that pressure can be applied to the pulmonary valve plate (PVP) under direct vision during the coring out procedure. By inflating the balloon (B), leakage of blood from the high-pressure right ventricle into the main pulmonary artery field after coring out is avoided.

Fig.3. The main pulmonary artery is opened longitudinally and the pulmonary valve plate (PVP) inspected. A 4- or 5-mm diameter coring device (D) has been most frequently used in this series of infants. Pressure from the ball-tipped probe (1 mm larger than coring device) below elevates the pulmonary valve plate and aligns it with the coring device. The coring device is rotated to make the cutout in the center of the valve plate (see insert). If blood obscures the main pulmonary artery field the balloon is inflated (through the handle) and pressed gently but firmly toward the remaining valve plate. S = Aortopulmonary shunt.

Fig.4. The anatomy of the heart following aortopulmonary shunt and core decompression is shown. The atrial septal defect is nonrestrictive following the balloon septostomy. The right ventricle has been decompressed by the core decompression and diastolic pressure has been reduced. Systolic pressure is often increased. A palpable thrill is usually present over the outflow tract (RVOT) of the right ventricle (RV) and blood flow to the lungs during this early post-coring phase still comes mainly from the aortopulmonary shunt (S). After several weeks the pulmonary blood flow will be increased by a greater contribution from the enlarging right ventricular chamber. Pulmonary diastolic murmurs are heard usually for the first time only several weeks after the core decompression.

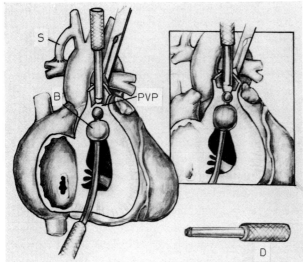

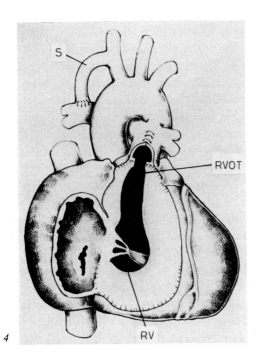

require ductus division to gain adequate distal control during the coring process. Large sutures (No. 2) may be passed around the proximal right and left pulmonary arteries or the distal MPA dissected free enough for a single cross-clamp to be applied. A purse string suture is placed on the RV just cephalad to the tricuspid valve on the RV and near the AV groove. 50 U of heparin per kilogram body weight are given at this time.

Since pinhole openings in the pulmonary valve plate are sometimes present but not seen on the initial angiogram (case 3), it is wise to gently squeeze out the MPA and occlude it distally. If the MPA refills, there must be a small communication from the RV to the MPA and the balloon backed ball tip device should be placed into the RV before opening the MPA. Usually there is no pinhole opening.

With distal MPA control maintained for 1 or 2 min to be sure cardiac output and O_2 saturation have not been compromised, the MPA is opened longitudinally and the valve plate inspected. It usually lies at an angle and will be better seen when pushed gently up from below with the ball tip. A running prolene stuture is placed so traction at each end will close the pulmonary arteriotomy quickly if needed. This suture is retracted out of the way (fig. 2).

A 4- or 5-mm coring device is selected depending on the pulmonary annulus size. At least a 2-mm rim of valve plate should remain after coring so that a good functional pulmonary valve will subsequently develop. The balloon backed ball tip device is selected 1 mm larger than the coring device. A No. 15 scalpel is used to create a stab wound through the RV purse string. A high pressure jet of dark blood should result or one may not have reached the real RV cavity. Endocardial fibroelastosis can make the endocardial layer difficult to penetrate. Once the ball tip and non-inflated balloon are in the RV, the purse string is cinched with a tourney and the ball tip advanced up to the valve plate.

The next few steps should be done quickly with the concept of minimum balloon inflation time and a clean *central* core of the valve plate removed. With ball tip pressure from below by the surgeon who also applies the coring device, rotation of the coring device placed at the center of the valve plate will cut away a 4- to 5-mm circular piece of the plate. If blood comes up from below, an assistant inflates the balloon with air until it stops (fig. 3). The coring device and the ball tip are kept pressed together and advanced into the MPA. Remove the coring device and cut free any final attachments of the circular piece of plate if needed. Fill the MPA with saline, pull on the prolene to close the MPA and immediately deflate the balloon. Release the distal MPA control, wait for a few heart beats to put aortic blood into the left lung then slowly remove the balloon-backed ball tip. There should be a 'pop' felt as the valve plate is crossed, and in all our cases a fine systolic thrill has been present at the pulmonary artery annulus. Closure is routine. The pericardium is closed except over the upper ascending aorta, and a right angle intrapericardial tube is placed between the heart and the diaphragm (fig. 4).

Total Open Heart Repair

The surgical procedure for the final open heart repair is similar to the repair of a tetralogy of Fallot without a ventricular septal defect (fig. 5). The essential steps are (1) pulmonary valvulotomy and valvuloplasty, (2) resection of the marked right ventricular outflow tract obstruction which in contrast to the tetralogy of Fallot leads up to and is confluent with the newly developed pulmonary valve, (3) closure of the ASD, and (4) closure of the aortopulmonary shunt. The tricuspid valve has not been approached or manipulated during the repair and neither stenosis or insufficiency has been found in postoperative follow-up (fig. 6).

Results

Initial Catheterization

The data obtained from the initial cardiac catheterizations are shown in table III. In all cases RV pressure exceeded the corresponding LV pressure. When an interatrial pressure gradient was found an atrial septostomy was done (3 cases). A patent ductus was demonstrable by angiography in 5 infants and not demonstrable in 2. High right atrial pressures found in 5 infants correlated well with large livers found on admission physical examinations. Arterial oxygen saturations varied with the degree of patency of the ductus. Of particular importance was the consistent finding of elevated RV end-diastolic pressures. Tricuspid insufficiency was present in all but 1 patient at angiography. It was mild in 4 infants and moderate in 2; these 2 had the lowest RV diastolic pressures.

We agree with others [1, 20, 21] that there is a continuous spectrum of RV size in patients with pulmonary atresia or pinhole pulmonary stenosis and an intact ventricular septum. Clinically most important is whether the chamber can manage a continuous stroke volume which is compatible with an adequate cardiac output and sustain life. We clinically classify chamber

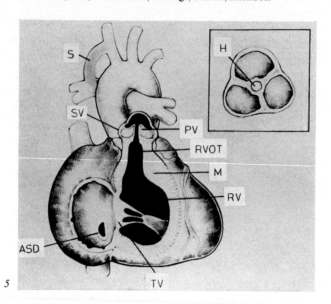

5

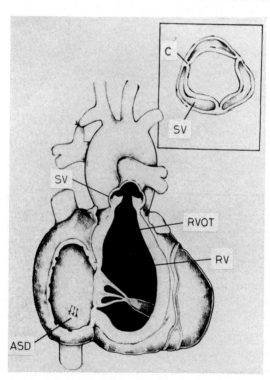

6

Table III. Initial cardiac catheterization data

Case No.	Weight, kg	HB	PDA	Arterial saturation, %	RAP	RVP	LVP	TI	Initial diagnosis
1	2.4	18.0	yes	59	15	75/30	70/20	+	PA c̄ IVS hypo. RV
2	2.4	19.2	no	30	15	85/30	60/15	+	PA c̄ IVS hypo. RV
3	3.9	19.0	no	30	25	100/25	64/18	+	PA c̄ IVS[1] hypo. RV
4	3.0	19.6	yes	82	20	110/25	75/15	0	PA c̄ IVS small RV
5	3.5	25.6	yes	79	8	90/10	40/10	+ +	PA c̄ IVS small RV
6	3.4	25.0	yes PGE$_1$	78	15	100/15	57/13	+	PA c̄ IVS small RV
7	3.7	18.6	yes PGE$_1$	70	5	145/5	140/0	+ +	crit. PS hypo. RV

PDA = latent ductus arteriosus; RAP = right arterial pressure; RVP = right ventricular pressure; LVP = left ventricular pressure; TI = tricuspid insufficiency; PA = pulmonary atresia; IVS = intact ventricular septum; RV = right ventricle; PS = pulmonary stenosis.
[1] Eccentric pinhole found in pulmonary valve plate at core decompression.

Fig. 5. At the time of total repair the intracardiac anatomy has changed significantly. The aortopulmonary shunt (S) remains patent, and the atrial septal defect (ASD) is relatively smaller and contributing little to cardiac output from the left heart. The right ventricular chamber (RV) has enlarged and the tricuspid annulus (TV) is somewhat larger than it was previously. There is significant infundibular muscular hypertrophy of the outflow tract (RVOT) of the right ventricle. These muscles (M) go all the way to the base of the pulmonary valve in contrast to the infundibular chamber of the typical tetralogy of Fallot. We have found a functional pulmonary valve (PV) has developed in the area of the original flat pulmonary plate in all cases. This change has included the development of sinuses of Valsalva (SV). The hole (H) in the valve has remained the same size as the device used during the original core decompression. Insert shows view of valve as seen from the main pulmonary artery.

Fig. 6. At the time of total repair the aortopulmonary shunt is closed, the pulmonary artery is opened and a pulmonary valvotomy is performed. In all 7 cases after total repair the pulmonary annulus has accommodated a 12-mm dilator with ease following the valvotomy. The commissures are taken down for 2 or 3 mm from their attachments to the pulmonary wall. The right ventricle (RV) is opened high in the outflow tract (RVOT) and the massive infundibular musculature resected to the base of the pulmonary valve in order to provide complete relief of the outflow tract obstruction from the right ventricle. The right atrium is then opened and the small atrial septal defect (ASD) closed with direct sutures. Note the significant change of pulmonary valve configuration from the time of initial valve plate coring to the time of total definitive repair, as shown in the insert. SV = Sinuses of Valsalva; C = commissures.

size into four categories: (1) hypoplastic: definitely unable to support an adequate cardiac output; (2) small: unable to support an adequate cardiac output but slightly larger than category 1; (3) medium: questionably able to sustain an adequate cardiac output; (4) large: normal or near normal size and able to sustain an adequate cardiac output.

All these patients fell into either category 1 (4 cases) or 2 (3 cases). In the total group of 23 patients any patient who was completely repaired with only a shunt before total repair was classified as a medium-sized RV or larger. Core decompression was reserved only for those cases which needed RV enlargement before a total repair could be accomplished.

Shunt and Core Decompression

The aortopulmonary shunt established satisfactory arterial O_2 saturations in all patients (range 66–89% saturation). The use of prostaglandin E_1 made the anesthesia and surgery much more stable, avoiding the acidosis and hypoxic episodes so common in the first 5 patients in this series.

The addition of core-decompression to the aortopulmonary shunt did not initially change arterial saturation, but as the RV enlarged with time and RV stroke volumes increased, the O_2 saturations did increase prior to final repair in each patient (range 81–94% saturation).

Core decompression did not alter RV systolic pressures. However, it did significantly lower RV end-diastolic pressure (fig. 7). As months passed after core decompression there was a small and statistically insignificant tendency for the RV systolic pressure to rise. RV end-diastolic pressure remained within normal limits until final open repair was accomplished in all patients.

Serial cardiac catheterizations and echocardiography permitted us to estimate RV growth and pulmonary valve development with time following core decompression (fig. 8). While the number of patients are too small for group comparisons, it did appear clinically that the initially small RV enlarged more rapidly than the initially hypoplastic RV (fig. 9). In all cases there was an increase in RV size, both in absolute volume and in comparison to left LV dimensions as described previously in the literature [1, 7, 8, 11, 17, 18, 21]. Every patient enlarged their RV to a size which was considered on clinical grounds adequate to maintain total cardiac output. When this point was reached, they were ready for the final open repair. The time from core decompression to final repair ranged from 23 to 44 months.

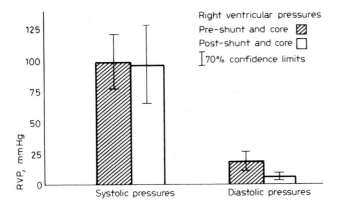

Fig. 7. Core decompression following an aortopulmonary shunt does not influence peak right ventricular systolic pressure (RVP). It does significantly (p < 0.01) reduce right ventricular end-diastolic pressure which then remains at normal levels as chamber size and valve anatomy develop.

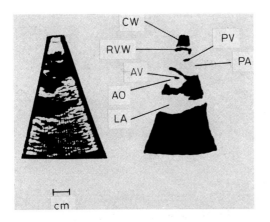

Fig. 8. Sector scanner, short axis plane 12 months following aortopulmonary shunt and core decompression. The scan demonstrates both aortic (AV) and pulmonary valves (PV) during ventricular diastole. The pulmonary artery (PA) is slightly larger than the aorta (AO) at this level. LA = Left atrium; RVW = right ventricular wall; CW chest wall.

Total Open Repair

Total open repair was accomplished in all 7 patients. Table IV and figure 10 show the pre- and postoperative data concerning RV pressures and pulmonary artery pressures along with follow-up EKG changes. The 1 death occurred a week following surgery in patient 4 who died of an overwhelming

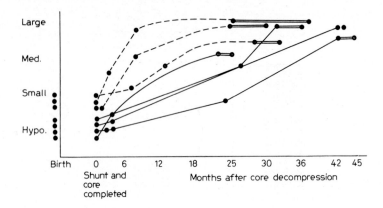

Fig. 9. Each point represents a cardiac catheterization and echo study evaluating right ventricular size and pulmonary valve development. Double lines depict the time interval between the last catheterization and the open total repair. Small ventricles (dashed lines) appeared to increase in size somewhat more rapidly than the hypoplastic right ventricles (solid lines).

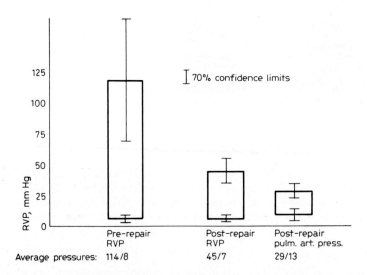

Fig. 10. Total open repair reduced peak right ventricular systolic pressures (RVP) from systemic levels to less than 50% of systemic levels in all 7 cases. Pulmonary artery pressures remained near normal. The mean right ventricular to pulmonary artery peak pressure gradient dropped from 84 to 16 mm Hg (p < 0.001).

Table IV Results of final open total repair PA c IVS and RV hypoplasia

	RV pressures			Flectrocardiogram	
Case No.	pre	post	PAP-post	pre-repair	follow-up post-repair
1	130/10	45/7	32/14	↑ RVH, RAH	WNL
2	210/5	36/5	30/12	↑ RVH, RAH	↓ RVH
3	75/10	60/10	40/20	↑ RVH, RAH	WNL
4	115/5	46/6	28/13	died: pulmonary syncytial virus 1 week postoperative	
5	90/7	50/5	25/12	↑ RVH, RAH	↓ RVH
6	135/8	55/10	25/12	↑ RVH, RAH	↓ RVH
7	45/5	27/10	25/10	RAH	WNL

PAP = Pulmonary artery pressure;   WNL = within normal limits; for further abbreviations see tables I–III.

Table V. Clinical status following open total Repair

Case No.	Duration of follow-up	Physical limitations	Tricuspid insufficiency	Pulmonary insufficiency grade	Medications
1	5 years	none	0	1	none
2	4 years	none	0	1	none
3	4 years	none	0	1	none
4	died: 1 week postoperative: pulmonary syncytial virus				
5	15 months	none	0	1	none
6	10 months	none	0	0	none
7	1 year	none	0	2	none

pulmonary viral infection. Postmortem examination showed massive pulmonary destruction, and cultures from the lungs and other body tissues grew dense populations of pulmonary syncytial virus. Bacterial cultures showed normal flora.

Subsequent patient follow-up is detailed in table V. None of the 6 survivors have any physical limitations. There is no evidence of tricuspid stenosis or insufficiency. None take any medications. All have soft systolic outflow tract murmurs, 4 have a grade 1 distolic murmur at the left upper sternal border and 1 has a grade 2 diastolic murmur there. 6 has no evidence of pulmonary insufficiency. EKGs show resolving RV hypoplasia or normal RV forces in all 6 patients.

Discussion

In the past the results of surgical repair in patients with pulmonary atresia and an intact ventricular septum who present in the newborn period have been dismal. Of 175 patients treated by a variety of surgical approaches reported between 1970 and 1978, 144 died either at the initial operation or during subsequent further surgery [2, 7–9, 11, 12]. This is a mortality rate of 82%. Although this is better than the 100% mortality in untreated patients [2], a trial of an alternative approach seemed warranted.

The newborn with pulmonary atresia and an intact ventricular septum needs: (1) increased pulmonary blood flow to relieve severe hypoxia; (2) a nonrestrictive ASD to handle the systemic venous return as cardiac output increases following an aortopulmonary shunt; (3) decompression of the RV to avoid arrhythmias and permit an increase in stroke volume capability, (4) time to modify the RV volume and pulmonary valve anatomy so as to permit a complete anatomical repair later in life.

Previous surgical approaches to pulmonary atresia with an intact ventricular septum have been limited because they were unable to consistently decompress the RV and maintain adequate pulmonary blood flow [8]. Many infants died despite a technically adept pulmonary valvotomy. Therefore, our first surgical procedure has been to create an aortopulmonary shunt to increase the pulmonary flow and to relieve the hypoxia. An ASD is important when the RV is small, but less important after the RV volume capacity has increased and the RV outflow tract has been decompressed.

Since a blind valvotomy has not been uniformly successful in decompressing the RV, a more consistently adequate technique was devised (fig. 2–4). This 'core decompression' technique permits direct visualization of the pulmonary valve plate during the coring procedure. In addition, counter pressure from the RV chamber insures correct alignment for the coring device to resect the specimen. We now realize that precise centering of the core-cutting device on the valve plate permits subsequent hemodynamic factors to mold a very satisfactory pulmonary valve and develop sinuses of Valsalva where none existed before.

The most significant early hemodynamic change caused by core decompression is diastolic pressure unloading of the RV. Forward blood flow from the RV into the pulmonary bed in hypoplastic or small RV cases may not be adequate to maintain cardiac output in the early post-core decompression period. 1 infant (from the group of 23) died when the Blalock shunt was injured during a CVP catheter insertion following a technically success-ful core decompression.

The murmur of pulmonary insufficiency, evidence of increased pul-monary blood flow and increasing volume handling ability of the RV, has been heard only several weeks after core decompression and is not associated with a reduction in peak RV systolic pressure. Pulmonary insufficiency and diastolic unloading appear to have the greatest influence on increasing RV volume.

The time course of hemodynamic alterations in the RV and pulmonary valve are not completely known. The urgency at the time of initial diagnosis and surgery makes a methodical evaluation of baseline chamber size and valve plate configuration difficult. Yet, it is clinically important that the time course be well documented so that appropriate clinical decisions can be made for future infants with this defect. It seems unlikely that we must wait for total repair until RV pressures reach dangerously high peak systolic levels. Valve plate molding into a functional valve occurred in patient 3 with relatively low RV pressures. It appears that flow may be the major deter-minant of valvular development and anatomy rather than systolic pressure.

Most of the current surgical approaches to pulmonary atresia and a hypoplastic RV with an intact ventricular septum still leave the patient with significant anatomical and hemodynamic limitations [5]. A few have been totally repaired using artificial valves and/or prosthetic conduits [19]. Late deaths and the potential need for further surgery occur in many cases. By allowing the pulmonary valve plate and the RV to develop to their intended anatomy and chamber size, the core decompression approach as seen in these 7 patients should significantly improve the long-term outlook for these patients. RV to pulmonary artery gradients were low following total open repair. In all cases RV:LV pressure ratios were less than 0.5. Follow-up electrocardiograms show that 3 of the 6 survivors have normal RV forces and all the others continue to move steadily in the same direction (table IV, V).

The findings and results in these patients have application to other complex forms of congenital heart disease, such as the hypoplastic left heart syndrome. We have learned that the potential for alteration of basic intra-cardiac chamber and valvular anatomy does not end at birth. Significant modification of the anatomy of congenital heart lesions can be accomplished given time and appropriate surgical manipulation of intracardiac hemo-dynamics shortly after birth, perhaps some day even before birth. Such surgical manipulations may make total anatomic repair of the defect possible at a later date.

References

1 Bowman, F.O.; Malm, J.R.; Haynes, C.J.; Gersony, W.M.; Ellis, K.: Pulmonary atresia with intact ventricular septum. J.thorac.cardiovasc.Surg.*61:* 85 (1971).

2 Buckley, L.P.; Dooley, K.J.; Fyler, D.C.: Pulmonary atresia and intact ventricular septum in New England. Am.J.Cardiol.*37:* 124 (1976).

3 Fyler, D.C.; Buckley, L.P.; Hellenbrand, W.E.; Cohn, H.E.: Report of the New England Regional Infant Cardiac Program. Pediatrics, Springfield *65:* suppl., p.450 (1980).

4 Trusler, G.A.; Fowler, R.S.: The surgical management of pulmonary atresia with intact ventricular septum and hypoplastic right ventricle. J.thorac.cardiovasc.Surg. *59:* 740 (1970).

5 Starr, A.: Critical pulmonary outflow obstruction with intact ventricular septum in neonates; in Parenzan, L.; Crupi, G.; Graham, G., Congenital heart disease in the first 3 months of life, p.535 (Patron Editore, Bologna 1981).

6 Gersony, W.M.; Bernhard, W.F.; Nadas, A.S.; Gross, R.E.: Diagnosis and surgical treatment of infants with critical pulmonary outflow obstruction. Circulation *35:* 765 (1967).

7 Ellis, K.; Casarella, W.J.; Hayes, C.J.; Gersony, W.M.; Bowman, F.O.; Malm, J.R.: Pulmonary atresia with intact ventricular septum. Am.J.Roentg. *116:* 501–513 (1972).

8 Moller, J.H.; Girod, D.; Amplatz, K.; Varco, R.L.: Pulmonary valvotomy in pulmonary atresia with hypoplastic right ventricle. Surgery, St Louis *68:* 630 (1970).

9 Trusler, G.A.; Yamamoto, N.; Williams, W.G.; Izukawa, T.; Rowe, R.D.; Mustard, W.T.: Surgical treatment of pulmonary atresia with intact ventricular septum. Br.Heart J. *38:* 957 (1976).

10 Luckstead, E.F.; Mattioli, L.; Crosby, I.K.; Reed, W.A.; Diehl, A.M.: Two-stage palliative surgical approach for pulmonary atresia with intact ventricular septum (type I). Am.J.Cardiol.*29:* 490 (1972).

11 Graham, T.P.; Bender, H.W.; Atwood, G.F.; Page, D.L.; Seli, C.G.R.: Increase in right ventricular volume following valvotomy for pulmonary atresia or stenosis with intact ventricular septum. Circulation *49/50:* 11–69 (1974).

12 Dhanavaravibul, S.; Nora, J.J.; McNamara, D.G.: Pulmonary valvular atresia with intact ventricular septum: problems in diagnosis and results of treatment. J.Pediat.*7:* 1010 (1970).

13 Shams, A.; Fowler, R.S.; Trusler, G.A.; Keith, J.D.; Mustard, W.T.: Pulmonary atresia with intact ventricular septum: report of 50 cases. Pediatrics, Springfield *47:* 370 (1971).

14 Greenwold, W.E.; DuShane, J.W.; Burchell, H.B.; et. al.: Congenital pulmonary atresia with intact ventricular septum: two anatomic types. Proceedings 29th Scientific Sessions, Circulation *14:* 9–15 (1956).

15 Avrom, K.V.; Edwards, J.E.: Relationship between right ventricular muscle bundles and pulmonary valve. Cardiovasc.Surg.*54:* suppl.111, pp.78–83 (1976).

16 Cole, R.B.; Muster, A.J.; Lev, M.; Paul, M.H.: Pulmonary atresia with intact ventricular septum. Am.J.Cardiol.*21:* 23 (1968).

17 Rao, P.S.; Liebman, J.; Borkat, G.: Right ventricular growth in a case of pulmonic

stenosis with intact ventricular septum and hypoplastic right ventricle. Circulation *53:* 389 (1976).

18   Free, M.D.; Rosenthal, A.; Bernhard, W.F.; Litwin, S.B.; Nadas, A.S.: Critical pulmonary stenosis with a diminutive right ventricle in neonates. Circulation *48:* 875 (1973).

19   Moulton, A.L.; Bowman, F.O., Jr.; Edie, R.N.; Hayes, C.J.; et al.: Pulmonary atresia with intact ventricular septum. J.thorac.cardiovasc.Surg. *78:* 527–537 (1979).

20   Zuberbuhler, J.R.; Anderson, R.H.: Morphological variations in pulmonary atresia with intact ventricular septum. Br. Heart J. *41:* 281–288 (1979).

21   Patel, R.G.; Freedom, R.M.; Moes, C.A.F.; et. al: Right ventricular volume determinations in 18 patients with pulmonary atresia and intact ventricular septum. Circulation *61:* 428 (1980).

Peter B.Mansfield, MD, Department of Surgery, Children's Orthopedic Hospital and Medical Center, P.O. Box C5371, Seattle, WA 98105 (USA)

Mod. Probl. Paediat., vol. 22, pp. 186–201 (Karger, Basel 1983)

Pulmonary Atresia with Ventricular Septal Defect

Fergus J. Macartney

Department of Paediatric Cardiology, The Hospital for Sick Children, London, England

Complete investigation of patients with pulmonary atresia with ventricular septal defect takes a lot of time, but is essential. Numerous angiograms are normally needed in order to demonstrate each abnormal anatomical detail, and this may result in overdosage with contrast medium and X-rays. The way to avoid this is to use angiography where it is essential (to demonstrate collateral circulation, and intrapulmonary artery anatomy), and to use two-dimensional echocardiography as far as possible to demonstrate the cardiac anatomy. For example, there is no need for left ventriculography in infants with complex pulmonary atresia, since primary intracardiac repair would not be contemplated at that age. Equally, there is no need to fill the whole of the right ventricle with contrast medium. Injections made into the right ventricle should be made with the catheter in the right ventricular outflow tract, using a relatively low dose of contrast medium. The reason for such an injection is simply to document whether there is actually complete pulmonary atresia, or severe tetralogy of Fallot, because the latter can mimic pulmonary atresia with ventricular septal defect, by presenting with little or no systolic murmur, and the continuous murmurs of major aortopulmonary collateral arteries.

Two-dimensional echocardiography will also demonstrate atrioventricular connections other than the concordant connection which is the rule in pulmonary atresia with ventricular septal defect, such as double inlet ventricle, and atrioventricular discordance.

When this policy of selected use of angiocardiography is adopted, the investigation of the patient remains technically demanding, but remarkably safe, since the only real way in which the patient can be harmed by extracardiac catheter manipulation is if an attempt is made to cross the *only* source of source of blood supply to the lungs, such as a patent ductus arteriosus. For this reason, the safest approach in the patient who has not previously been investigated is to carry upper descending aortography (fig. 1) as the first stage of angiocardiographic investigation, prior to attempting entry to collateral arteries or central pulmonary arteries with the catheter. This procedure will demonstrate patency of any normally positioned ductus arteriosus (fig. 2), as well as the great majority of major aortopulmonary collateral arteries. A similar, but occasionally superior angiocardiogram is obtained if a balloon is floated through the heart and aorta to lie in the lower descending thoracic aorta. While the aorta is temporarily occluded with the inflated balloon, contrast medium is injected through side holes proximal to the balloon (fig. 3).

Injection of contrast medium into the aortic root or one of the ventricles is only necessary, as far as demonstration of pulmonary blood supply is concerned, if there is reason to suspect that it has not all been demonstrated on the descending aortogram. Comparison of the downstream injection in the upper descending aorta, and the upstream injection, will permit recognition of the rarer natural communications between aorta and pulmonary artery, such as coronary artery/pulmonary artery fistula, aortopulmonary window, persistent ductus contralateral to the aortic arch (fig. 4), anomalous origin of one pulmonary artery from the ascending aorta, or other major collateral arteries from the brachiocephalic arteries. Aortopulmonary window, persistent ductus contralateral to the aortic arch, and anomalous origin of one pulmonary artery from the ascending aorta have all recently been shown to be fairly easily diagnosable by cross-sectional echocardiography [Smallhorn et al., 1982a, b].

Ideally, all injections made to demonstrate the sources of pulmonary blood supply are carried out in the same projection, since detailed analysis will usually consist of comparison of several different angiograms. If the equipment is such that caudo-cranial tilt can be produced without moving the patient, we would use the combination of a frontal projection with caudo-cranial tilt, and a standard lateral projection. Otherwise, standard frontal and lateral projections are best.

Selective Injections into Central Pulmonary Arteries,
Surgical Shunts and Collateral Arteries

Manipulation of transvenous catheters passed through the heart into the aorta enables most of the sites necessary for selective angiograms to be

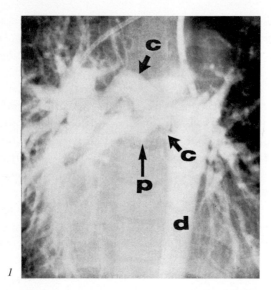

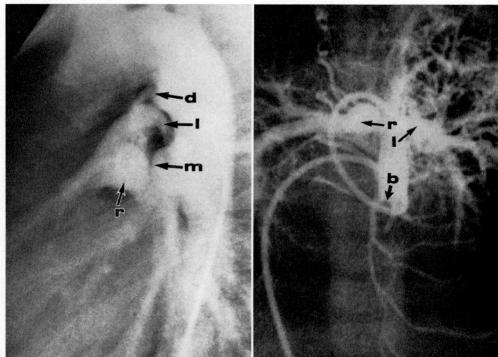

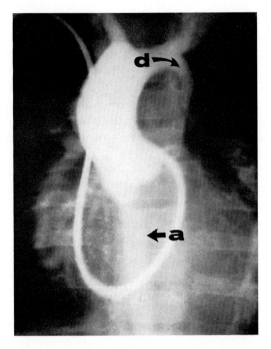

Fig.4. Frontal plane, ascending aortogram. Note that there is a right aortic arch as indicated by the position of the descending aorta (a). A patent ductus arteriosus (d) originates just proximal to the bifurcation of the innominate artery, which is on the left.

Fig.1. Frontal view of upper descending aortogram. Note the descending aorta (d), the major aortopulmonary collateral arteries (c), and pulmonary trunk (p) bifurcating into the left and right pulmonary arteries.

Fig.2. Lateral projection, upper descending aortogram. Note the ductus arteriosus (d) supplying the left (1) and right (r) pulmonary arteries. Note also that there are major aortopulmonary collateral arteries, supplying in fact both right and left pulmonary arteries from a common trunk (m). In other words, both lungs are supplied both by a ductus arteriosus and by collaterals.

Fig.3. Frontal plane, descending aortogram using a balloon cathether. This patient had pulmonary atresia with intact septum and had previously had a left thoracotomy with formalin infiltration of the ductus arteriosus, which had subsequently closed spontaneously. The catheter has been advanced from the transvenous route and looped in the left ventricle to pass round the aortic arch. Note the balloon (b), which completely occludes the descending aorta. From the descending aorta, an incredibly dense plexus of acquired collateral arises, particularly on the left, which opacifies the central left (1) and right (r) pulmonary arteries.

reached, but usually not all. In the end, it is usually quicker to use the retro-grade arterial route, unless one is concerned about complications of arterial catheterization in babies. From the axillary artery, collateral arteries are a little harder to enter, but once they are entered, with flexible tipped catheters, such as a Sones coronary artery catheter or a Shirey transvalvular catheter, it is easier to pass a long way down a collateral into the intrapulmonary or even central pulmonary arteries. However, percutaneous catheterization of the femoral artery is the most generally applicable technique, and will there-fore be the one described.

Our preference is to use pre-curved catheters of cobra shape, with or without end holes, depending on whether a guidewire is likely to be used. The long curve of the neck of the cobra keeps its head (the tip) pressed against the wall of the aorta, so that the tip automatically enters any side branch of the descending aorta, including collateral arteries (fig. 5). The tight curve at the catheter tip is extremely valuable for crossing surgical shunts, particularly from the subclavian arteries. Once the tip is engaged in the shunt, a guide wire passed down it will traverse the length of the shunt and enter the central pulmonary artery (fig. 6).

The tight curve on the end of the catheter also may permit the other-wise impossible entry to the proximal right pulmonary artery from a Waterston shunt. The tip of the catheter is passed through the anastomosis and directed leftward. Then either a straight or J-wire is passed through the ca-theter, so as to travel retrograde down the proximal right pulmonary artery.

It is almost always possible to enter the central pulmonary artery when a previous surgical shunt has been constructed. Occasionally, it is possible to achieve the same through a natural major aortopulmonary collateral, though this manoeuvre is often frustrated by the tortuosity of such arteries. If the central pulmonary artery can be entered, or a catheter can be passed well down the collateral artery or shunt supplying the central pulmonary artery, a selective injection is best shot in the right and left anterior oblique projections, since this provides more accurate assessment of which segments of the two lungs are connected to the central pulmonary arteries. The dis-advantage of frontal and lateral projections of such angiograms in this particular instance is the overlapping between the two lungs in the lateral projection, which makes it impossible to distinguish between the left and right lung. Simultaneous injection into the rigth ventricular outflow tract and pulmonary artery (fig. 6, 7) neatly demonstrates the extent of the 'gap' between the blind ends of the right ventricular outflow tract and pulmonary trunk [*Freedom* et al., 1974], though this is not all that important.

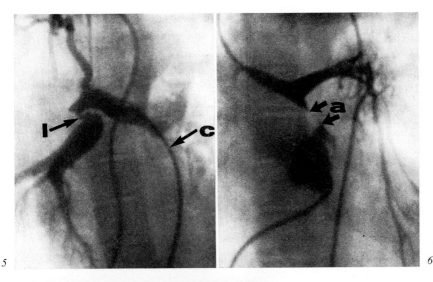

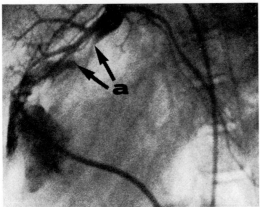

Fig.5. Frontal projection, selective injection into major aortopulmonary collateral in same patient as figure 1, but following a right thoracotomy with ligation of one major aortopulmonary collateral artery immediately proximal to the point (1) and creation of a right Blalock-Taussig anastomosis. The cobra shaped catheter (c) sits nicely in the collateral artery, which since its ligation has developed two branches which were not previously present, one running upwards, and the other (1) communicating with the right lower lobe pulmonary artery.

Fig.6. Frontal projection angiocardiogram from same patient as illustrated in figures 1 and 5. One catheter has been advanced through a Blalock-Taussig anastomosis into the pulmonary trunk, and the other placed in the right ventricular outflow tract. By simultaneous injection, the extent of atresia (a) has been demonstrated.

Fig.7. Lateral projection of figure 6. Note the demonstrated atretic segment (a).

Hand injection of contrast medium is usually adequate for demonstration of smaller collateral arteries, but power injection is preferable in large collaterals otherwise the considerable blood flow will produce excessive dilution of contrast medium.

During manipulation to enter major aortopulmonary collateral arteries originating from the descending aorta, intercostal arteries are frequently entered (fig. 8) particularly because they may be enlarged as a result of supplying acquired collateral circulation to the lungs. Entry to an intercostal artery may be suspected from the posterior course of the catheter from the aorta towards the paravertebral gutter. In contrast, major aortopulmonary collateral arteries pass anterior from the aorta towards the hilum (fig. 2). When contrast medium is injected into an intercostal artery, the patient often complains of burning pain in the intercostal muscles, but no other harm appears to result.

Catheters should always be passed as far distal into any collateral as possible in order to document pressure gradients in vessels. These are not always accompanied by an angiographic stenosis [Macartney et al., 1973].

Pulmonary Wedge Angiography

Using selective injections into major aortopulmonary collateral arteries, it is almost invariably possible to demonstrate central pulmonary arteries [Haworth and Macartney, 1980]. Only if these methods fail to demonstrate central pulmonary arteries would we resort to pulmonary vein wedge angiography [Nihill et al., 1978; Singh et al., 1978]. Serious complications of this technique have been described with power injections, including perforation of the bronchial wall by contrast medium [Alpert and Culham. 1979]. We therefore recommend the technique suggested by Nihill et al. [1948]. An end hole catheter is wedged in a pulmonary vein. 0.5 ml/kg of contrast medium are then injected by hand, immediately followed by 1 ml/kg of 5 % dextrose. If the first injection is successful, contrast medium is forced back through the pulmonary capillaries and intrapulmonary arteries into the hilum of the lung, whence the central pulmonary arteries and other intrapulmonary arteries may then opacify. Injection of dextrose continues this process, and then clears the 'smudge' of contrast medium in the injection site.

Our experience is that even with good technique, a single pulmonary venous wedge angiogram frequently fails to demonstrate central pulmonary arteries even when they are present. This seems to be for one of three reasons.

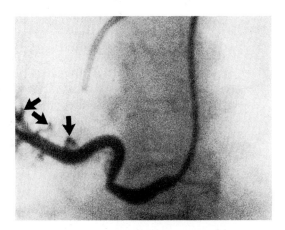

Fig.8. Frontal projection, selective right intercostal arteriogram. Note the multiple small acquired collaterals (arrows) originating from the intercostal artery and spreading into the parietal pleura, from which anastomoses with the visceral pleural will permit the creation of acquired systemic pulmonary collateral circulation.

Firstly, blood flow through the central pulmonary arteries may be in the wrong direction. For example, if flow is from left pulmonary artery to right, even if contrast medium is forced back from the right pulmonary veins to a right hilar artery connected to the central pulmonary artery, that artery may still not opacify. Secondly, the hilar vessel opacified may not be connected to the central pulmonary arteries. Finally, the pressure in the artery which supplies the vessel into which the catheter is wedged may be so high that it is impossible to force contrast medium backwards against the current. Thus, it is necessary to perform pulmonary venous wedge angiography in multiple sites in order to exclude the presence of a central pulmonary artery. In short, pulmonary venous wedge angiography works best when one low pressure central pulmonary artery is connected to all the hilar arteries in one lung. One rare reason for this is interruption of a central pulmonary artery, which can be either congenital or else unintentionally acquired due to unsuccessful surgery. Under these circumstances, there may be no large vessels connected to the pulmonary artery distal to the interruption, and attempts to demonstrate the pulmonary artery from the arterial side may well be unsuccessful. In our view, the only situation under which the basically unphysiological procedure of pulmonary vein wedge angiography is superior to selective injections on the arterial side of the circulation is that in which the entire pulmonary blood supply to one lung or both is acquired.

Angiographic Analysis

The following four questions need to be answered: (a) How does the blood reach the pulmonary circulation from the systemic circulation? (b) Is either or are both central pulmonary arteries present, and are they confluent? (c) How are the sources of pulmonary blood supply, the central pulmonary arteries, and the intrapulmonary arteries interconnected? (d) What obstructions exist in the system as a whole? These questions will be dealt with in turn.

Sources of pulmonary blood supply form a particularly good example of the use of applied embryology. For example, a persistent ductus arteriosus on the contralateral side from the aortic arch (fig. 4) is likely to originate close to the bifurcation of the innominate artery, and pass to the ipsilateral central pulmonary artery, usually taking a straight course, but sometimes 'wandering'. Rarely, the ductus may co-exist with major aortopulmonary collateral arteries, either one on one side and the other on the other or, occasionally, with both supplying both lungs (fig. 2) [*Macartney and Haworth*, 1982].

A persistent fifth aortic arch would be expected to course from the distal ascending aorta proximal to the first brachiocephalic artery to the central pulmonary artery, as described previously in a hitherto unique case [*Macartney* et al., 1974]. We believe we may have identified a second case of persistent fifth aortic arch in association with pulmonary atresia in a patient with interruption of the right pulmonary artery [*Macartney and Haworth*, 1982].

Major aortopulmonary collateral arteries appear as large tortuous arteries, rarely more than six in number, originating usually from the descending aorta (fig. 1, 2, 5), but occasionally from brachiocephalic arteries (fig. 9, 11) and exceptionally from coronary arteries [*Macartney* et al., 1973].

Major aortopulmonary collateral arteries anastomose with intrapulmonary arteries in the neighbourhood of the hilum and, unlike bronchial arteries, are never connected to intercostal arteries. They accompany bronchi, but never form a plexus round them and look essentially the same throughout life.

Acquired collateral circulation is, by contrast, extremely rare in the first 3 months of life, but becomes better and better developed with the passage of time, particular after thoracotomies, when adhesions between the visceral and parietal pleurae form pathways for acquired collateral circulation from the chest wall to the lungs (fig. 3, 11). When aortography is performed, ac-

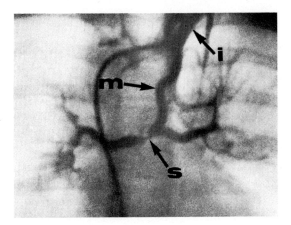

Fig. 9. Selective innominate artery (i) injection in a patient with pulmonary atresia with ventricular septal defect. Frontal projection. Note the major aortopulmonary collateral artery (m) originating from the innominate artery, giving off a branch to the left upper zone and then bifurcating to right and left, with a stenosis (s) of its right branch. This artery crossing the mediastinum is not the central pulmonary artery, which was demonstrated on another collateral artery injection to be grossly hypoplastic, and of the typical 'seagull' appearance.

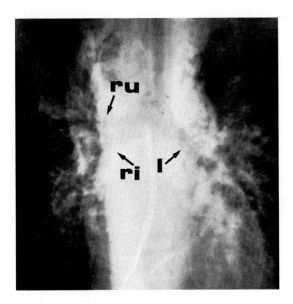

Fig. 10. Late frame of aortogram, reproduced by kind permission of Dr. *Jane Somerville.* Frontal projection. Note that the bronchial tree is highlighted by the plexus of bronchial arteries in the walls of the bronchi. ru = Right upper lobe bronchus; ri = right intermediate stem bronchus; l = left main bronchus.

quired collateral circulation appears as countless minute vessels originating from any artery in the thorax. Bronchial arteries can be recognized as such because of their close relation to the trachea and main bronchi, and the way in which they form a nutritive plexus in the bronchial wall. This plexus 'lights up' during an aortogram, because of the contrast between air in the lumen and contrast medium in the walls (fig. 10).

More detailed analysis of acquired collateral circulation can be obtained by selective injections into intercostal, coronary, or internal mammary arteries [*Macartney and Haworth*, 1982]. In contrast with major aorto-pulmonary collateral arteries, recognizable, discrete anastomoses within the pulmonary arteries in the region of the hilum are extremely rare.

Central pulmonary arteries are most easily recognized when they are confluent, as they usually are (fig. 1, 6). The confluent pulmonary arteries together with the hypoplastic pulmonary trunk resembles a seagull in flight in the frontal plane [*Somerville* et al., 1978]. Caudo-cranial tilt, by elongating the pulmonary trunk, accentuates the resemblance. In the lateral projection, the confluent central pulmonary arteries appear as a hairpin, extending anteriorly to the trachea [*Fäller* et al., 1981].

If there is doubt as to the nature of a mediastinal artery, it is helpful to view the cine angiogram in motion, because pulmonary arteries, being attached to the heart, tend to move with it, whereas collateral arteries, originating from the descending aorta and passing to the lung, tend to move with respiration [*Fäller* et al., 1981].

Interconnection between Central Pulmonary Arteries, Intrapulmonary Arteries and Collateral Arteries

In pulmonary atresia, as in almost all other congenital heart defects, the intrapulmonary arteries are, in essence, normal. In particular, with rare exceptions their intrapulmonary distribution is that of normal pulmonary arteries (fig. 5, 9). Such abnormalities as exist tend to reflect the haemo-dynamic conditions [*Macartney and Haworth*, 1979]. If collateral arteries are hypoperfused, and at low pressure, they look narrow, with deficient peripheral branching. If on the other hand they are hyperperfused and at high pressure, they appear large and tortuous, with increased background haze. When pulmonary vascular obstructive disease supervenes, background haze diminishes while the arteries remain tortuous.

The primary abnormalities of the intrapulmonary arteries are almost entirely confined to the hilum, where in most cases there is a 'connection problem' [*Haworth* et al., 1981b]. The intrapulmonary arteries, instead of being connected to a single hilar artery, in normal fashion, may remain quite separate. As a result, the pulmonary arterial supply to an entire lobe, or segment, or even part of a segment, may be completely isolated from the remainder of the lung (fig. 11). Proximally, the segmental or lobar arteries are connected either to a central pulmonary artery, to a major aortopulmonary collateral artery, or to both. The usual result is that pulmonary blood supply is strictly compartmentalized, and 'one-to-one' (fig. 12). In other words, each major aortopulmonary collateral artery supplies a unique region of lung. When contrast medium is injected into that major aortopulmonary collateral artery, one unique region of lung is opacified. However, we have recently recognized that when cine angiograms of selective injections into major aortopulmonary collateral arteries are reviewed, washout of contrast medium by non-opacified blood entering a particular point in an intrapulmonary artery is not infrequently seen. Likewise, some highly diluted contrast medium may wash in into an adjacent region of lung. Both of these appearances result from the fact that more than one major aortopulmonary collateral artery is supplying the same region of lung (fig. 12). We have dubbed this phenomenon duplicate pulmonary blood supply [*Fäller* et al., 1981].

When all the information from all selective injections is pooled, it should be possible to state precisely whence blood supply to each pulmonary segment originates and, most importantly, how much of the parenchyma of each lung is connected to each pulmonary artery. This is why it is important to recognize the existence of duplicate pulmonary blood supply. Otherwise, a misleading impression will be obtained. For example, suppose that the right upper lobe appears to be connected to a major aortopulmonary collateral artery *and* to the central right pulmonary artery, whereas the right lower lobe appears only to be connected to a major aortopulmonary collateral artery. At first site, a shunt into the central right pulmonary artery, or indeed a 'corrective' conduit operation, will only increase the blood supply to the right lower lobe. But if careful inspection reveals washin or washout from one lobe to the other, then such operations would actually provide a fresh source of pulmonary blood supply to the entire lung.

Obstructions to pulmonary blood supply may occur at the immediate site of the aortopulmonary anastomosis, within an aortopulmonary conduit, within the central pulmonary arteries, within the intrapulmonary arteries, or at arteriolar level.

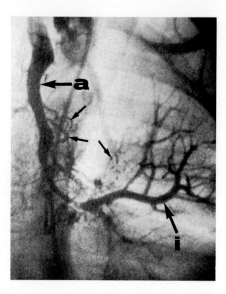

Fig. 11. Selective injection into major aortopulmonary collateral artery originating from the right subclavian artery. Frontal projection. Note the way the collateral is immediately adjacent to the aortic arch (a), and supplies intrapulmonary arteries (i) to a very limited region of the left lung. Note also the acquired collateral circulation to the left lung produced by a previous thoracotomy (multiple small arrows).

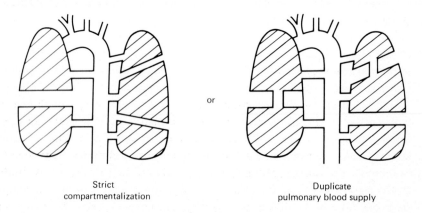

Strict
compartmentalization

or

Duplicate
pulmonary blood supply

Fig. 12. Diagram to illustrate the difference between strict compartmentalization and duplicate pulmonary blood supply. When there is strict compartmentalization there is one collateral artery for each region of lung supplied, i.e. a 'one-to-one' relationship. When pulmonary blood supply is duplicate, there are regions of lung which receive from two separate collaterals. In the diagram the right lung and the left upper zone have duplicate pulmonary blood supply, whereas the left lower zone has 'one-to-one' supply.

Obstruction within an aortopulmonary conduit is found in natural communications, such as major aortopulmonary collateral arteries (fig. 9), or a persistent ductus arteriosus (fig. 2), as well as the less common coronary artery/pulmonary artery fistulas [*Krongrad* et al., 1972], or a persistent fifth aortic arch [*Macartney* et al., 1974]. The same obstruction may be found in surgically created Blalock-Taussig shunts or synthetic conduits inserted between the aorta or subclavian arteries and the pulmonary arteries. Usually there is an abrupt pressure drop at the pulmonary end of the anastomosis [*Macartney* et al., 1974]. Rarely the pressure difference consists of a gradual change in pressure over the whole length of the conduit.

Obstruction within the central pulmonary arteries may be observed angiocardiographically [*McGoon* et al., 1977; *Macartney and Haworth*, 1979].

Obstruction at arteriolar level certainly occurs as classical pulmonary vascular obstructive disease secondary to hypertensive hyperperfusion, and tends to occur in segments or subsegments of lungs supplied by unobstructed major aortopulmonary collateral arteries [*Jefferson* et al., 1972; *Thiene* et al., 1979; *Haworth and Macartney*, 1980]. However, the changes due to hypoperfusion may have a more profound effect on pulmonary vascular resistance than has hitherto been imagined. In particular, intimal proliferation in acquired collateral circulation appears to extend into the pulmonary arteries within the acinus, at least in experimental animals [*Haworth* et al., 1981a]. This intimal proliferation would presumably raise pulmonary vascular resistance.

Decisions Regarding Surgery

The hospital mortality of correction of pulmonary atresia with ventricular septal defect closely relates to the postoperative ratio between the right and left systolic pressures. This ratio may be predicted from the body surface area, the relative diameters of the left and right pulmonary arteries and the aorta at the diaphragm, the presence of stenosis at the origin of the right pulmonary artery, and the presence of arborization anomalies, which correspond to the connection problem described above [*Alfieri* et al., 1978]. The formula produced by the quoted workers may be, and has been, criticized on three grounds. Firstly, the cross-sectional area of the pulmonary arteries is presumably of more importance than the diameter. Secondly, the formula takes no account of the pulmonary artery pressure. Thirdly, one should probably be trying to quantitate the amount of lung connected to central pulmonary arteries on a continuous scale, rather than simply defining it an arborization abnormality as being present or absent. However, no better alternative to this very imaginative piece of original work is currently available.

If the predicted ventricular systolic pressure ratio is above 0.75, corrective surgery should not be carried out, and we would favour a shunt operation with or without unifocalization [*Haworth* et al., 1981a, b; *Macartney* et al., 1982]. Even if the predicted pressure ratio is less than this figure, the correct decision may not be to proceed with immediate definitive repair. For example, it may be possible to get away in the short run with repair in a patient who has large central pulmonary arteries without correcting a severe arborization abnormality in one lung. However, had that arborization abnormality been corrected, either prior to or during definite surgery, it might well be that the long-term outlook of the patient would be better.

References

Alfieri, O.; Blackstone, E.H.; Kirklin, J.W.; Pacifico, A.D.; Bargeron, L.M., Jr.: Surgical treatment of tetralogy of Fallot with pulmonary atresia. J.thorac.cardiovasc.Surg. *76:* (1978) 321–335.

Alpert, B.S.; Culham, J.A.G.: A severe complication of pulmonary vein angiography. Br.Heart J. *41:* 727–729 (1979).

Fäller, K.; Haworth, S.G.; Taylor, J.F.N.; Macartney, F.J.: Duplicate sources of pulmonary blood supply in pulmonary atresia with ventricular septal defect. Br.Heart J. *46:* 263–268 (1981).

Freedom, R.M.; White, R.I., jr.; Ho, C.S.; Gingell, R.L.; Hawker, R.E.; Rowe, R.D.: Evaluation of patients with pulmonary atresia and intact ventricular septum by double catheter technique. Am.J.Cardiol. *33:* 892–895 (1974).

Haworth, S.G.; Leval, M. de; Macartney, F.J.: How the left lung is perfused after ligating the left pulmonary artery in the pig at birth: clinical implications for the hypoperfused lung. Cardiovasc.Res. *15:* 214–226 (1981a).

Haworth, S.G.; Macartney, F.J.: Growth and development of pulmonary circulation in pulmonary atresia with ventricular septal defect and major aortopulmonary collateral arteries. Br.Heart J. *44:* 14–24 (1980).

Haworth, S.G.; Rees, P.G.; Taylor, J.F.N.; Macartney, F.J.; Leval de, M.; Stark, J.: Pulmonary atresia with ventricular septal defect and major aortopulmonary collateral arteries. Effect of systemic pulmonary anastomosis. Br.Heart J. *45:* 133–141 (1981b).

Jefferson, K.; Rees, S.; Somerville, J.: Systemic arterial supply to the lungs in pulmonary atresia and its relation to pulmonary artery development. Br. Heart J. *34:* 418–427 (1972).

Krongrad, E.; Ritter, D.G.; Hawe, A.; Kincaid, O.W.; McGoon, D.C.: Pulmonary atresia or severe stenosis and coronary artery-to-pulmonary artery fistula. Circulation 46: 1005–1012 (1972).

Macartney, F.; Deverall, P.; Scott, O.: Haemodynamic characteristics of systemic arterial blood supply to the lungs. Br. Heart J. 35: 28–37 (1973).

Macartney, F.J.; Haworth, S.G.: The pulmonary blood supply in pulmonary atresia with ventricular septal defect; in Godman, Marquis, Paediatric cardiology, vol.2, pp. 314–338 (Churchill-Livingstone, Edinburgh 1979).

Macartney, F.J.; Haworth, S.G.: Investigation of pulmonary atresia with ventricular septal defect; in Anderson, Macartney, Shinebourne, Tynan, Paediatric cardiology, vol.5 (Churchill-Livingstone, Edinburgh in press, 1982).

Macartney, F.J.; Huhta, J.C.; Douglas, J.M.; Haworth, S.G.; Leval, M.R. de; Stark, J.: The long-term results of surgery for pulmonary atresia with ventricular septal defect. Cœur in press, 1982).

Macartney, F.J.; Scott, O.; Deverall, P.B.: Haemodynamic and anatomical characteristics of pulmonary blood supply in pulmonary atresia with ventricular septal defect – including a case of persistent fifth aortic arch. Br. Heart J. 36: 1049–1060 (1974).

McGoon, M.D.; Fulton, R.E.; Davis, G.D.; Ritter, D.G.; Neill, C.A.; White, R.I.: Systemic collateral and pulmonary artery stenosis in patients with congenital pulmonary valve atresia and ventricular septal defect. Circulation 56: 473–479 (1977).

Nihill, M.R.; Mullins, C.E.; McNamara, D.G.: Visualization of the pulmonary arteries in pseudotruncus by pulmonary vein wedge angiography. Circulation 58: 140–147 (1978).

Singh, S.P.; Righby, M.L.; Astley, R.: Demonstration of pulmonary arteries by contrast injection into pulmonary vein. Br. Heart J. 40: 55–57 (1978).

Smallhorn, J.F.; Anderson, R.H.; Macartney, F.J.: Two-dimensional echocardiographic assessment of communications between the ascending aorta and the pulmonary trunk or individual pulmonary arteries. Br. Heart J. 47: 563–572 (1982a).

Smallhorn, J.F.; Huhta, J.C.; Anderson, R.H.; Macartney, F.J.: Suprasternal cross-sectional echocardiography in assessment of patent ductus arteriosus. Br. Heart J. (in press, 1982b).

Somerville, J.; Saravalli, O.; Ross, D.: Complex pulmonary atresia with congenital systemic collaterals. Classification and management. Archs Mal Cœur 71: 322–328 (1978).

Thiene, G.; Frescura, C.; Bini, R.M.; Valente, M.; Gallucci, V.: Histology of pulmonary arterial supply in pulmonary atresia with ventricular septal defect. Circulation 60: 1066–1074 (1979).

Fergus J. Macartney, MD, Department of Paediatric Cardiology, The Hospital for Sick Children, Great Ormond Street, London WC1N 3JH (England)

Mod. Probl. Paediat., vol. 22, pp. 202–209 (Karger, Basel 1983)

Technique of Profound Hypothermia, Perfusion and Cardioplegia in Infant Surgery

G. A. Trusler

Department of Surgery, University of Toronto and the Hospital for Sick Children, Toronto, Ontario, Canada

In the 1950s, moderate hypothermia to approximately 30 °C was employed for the repair of simple cardiac defects. Attempts at using some form of deep hypothermia to correct more major defects were unsuccessful because surgical techniques were relatively primitive and cardiopulmonary bypass, used for cooling and rewarming, was associated with significant morbidity and mortality, particularly in infants where the potential advantages of a quiet dry operative field were most important. In the early 1960s, general interest in deep profound hypothermia dwindled, while operative techniques and cardiopulmonary bypass improved. However, later in the decade, a few surgeons including *Horiuchi* et al. [5], *Muraoka* et al. [8], *Barrett-Boyes* et al. [2] and *Mohri* et al. [7] started to use deep hypothermia in the repair of the heart defects. While much is not known about the effects of deep hypothermia, the usefulness of the technique is unquestioned. The relaxed still exposure obtained by hypothermic circulatory arrest has extended the capabilities of surgeons and simplified the application of even complex repairs to small infants.

Techniques

Profound Hypothermia

Between 1967 and December, 1980, 689 patients at the Hospital for Sick Children, Toronto, have had cardiac malformations repaired with profound hypothermia and circulatory arrest. Our first patients were described by *Bailey* et al. [1], and a later review was carried out by *Geiss* [unpublished]. The first 11 patients in this series underwent surface cooling alone to an average esophageal temperature of 20 °C, followed by circulatory stasis for intra-cardiac repair. Since June, 1969, deep hypothermia has been achieved by means of surface cooling to 25–28 °C (in the first 16 patients) or to 31–32 °C (in the subsequent 203 patients) prior to core (perfusion) cooling, to an esophageal temperature of 14–18 °C and rectal temperature of 20 °C or below. To obtain more myocardial protection, for the past 4–5 years, infants have been cooled to a rectal temperature between 15 and 18 °C in most cases. Following intracardiac repair, rewarming in all instances was accomplished by partial cardiopulmonary bypass and surface rewarming. At one time, a second period of circulatory arrest was used to provide the extended time necessary to repair complicated defects. Since this caused some cerebral complications and increased mortality, it was abandoned. 13 % of the patients had some period of interval hypothermic perfusion where the repair was prolonged, some at low flow and some at normal flow rates. It is important to realize that with bypass cooling, the esophageal temperature represents blood temperature. Rectal temperature is closer to that of the body mass, and is therefore a safer guide to the degree of general hypothermia and brain temperature.

An investigation by the members of our anesthetic staff headed by *Johnson* and *Steward* resulted in some modifications of the earlier technique [6].

(1) Because of significant decreases in plasma potassium concentration during the initial cooling in the first group of patients, and the possible relationship of this to ventricular fibrillation in digitalized patients, we started bypass cooling before the esophageal temperature reached 30 °C. Now there is no formal surface cooling but the child is allowed to cool spontaneously during induction of anesthesia, subsequent patient preparation and the early part of the operative procedure.

(2) The addition of 6.0 ml of 10 % calcium chloride and heparin per unit blood used in the oxygenator prime or as replacement during bypass, was required to maintain normal calcium ion activity.

(3) At one time, 10 % carbon dioxide was required to maintain an arterial CO_2 level of 40 mm Hg during the cooling bypass. Now with use of the membrane oxygenator relatively little CO_2 is added to maintain a level of 40 mm Hg. We feel this improves cerebral circulation and possibly myocardial rhythmicity.

(4) The postoperative dosage of potassium in these infants was increased to 3–4 mEq/kg/24 h for 1–2 days depending on the adequacy of renal function and plasma potassium concentrations.

(5) In 2 infants, deaths were considered to be related to a low serum magnesium. Consequently, magnesium has been administered post-operatively in a dosage of 1 mEq/kg/24 h, for 24 h.

Perfusion

The technique of perfusion is fairly simple. We use a single arterial cannula in the ascending aorta and, in most infants, a single venous cannula in the right atrium. Occasionally, in complicated cases where the repair takes longer than is safe with a single episode of circulatory arrest, part of the repair is done during perfusion with two venous cannulae. These cannulae are usually inserted through the atrial incision itself during a brief period of circulatory arrest. We use two acutely curved metal venous cannulae which provide good venous return. In certain situations, such as repair of truncus arteriosus, part of the repair is done during hypothermic low-flow perfusion and part with circulatory arrest, similar to the technique used by *Ebert* et al. [3].

Hypothermia low-flow bypass has been widely used to some degree for many years. By tailoring the degree of hypothermia and low-flow to the needs of the child, the blood damage from bypass is reduced. The operative field is quiet and cardiotomy return is easily controlled. When combined with circulatory arrest, it is a convenient way of reducing both circulatory arrest and full-flow bypass time.

Cardioplegia

For approximately 5 years, we have used cold potassium cardioplegia in infants and children to help preserve myocardial function and produce greater relaxation during circulatory arrest. We use the cardioplegic solution devised by *Roe* et al. [9] of San Francisco. This is administered by the anesthetist through an infusion line inserted into the root of the aorta using a No.16 or No.18 needle. The cardioplegic solution is cooled to 4°C and given in an amount equal to 300 ml/m² surface area and at a pressure of 150 mm Hg at source. At one time, the injection was repeated after 20–30 min of arrest but this is seldom done now because the heart remains cold and electrical activity does not return spontaneously. A trial of blood cardioplegia was abandoned because we found it difficult to control ionized serum calcium without suitable equipment. Many variations in the technique of delivery of cardioplegia have been described. The actual technique is not critical as long as the solution is given at a safe but adequate pressure and low temperature.

Other factors which contribute to the hypothermia technique include adequate operating room air conditioning and an improved lighting system which produces less radiant heat on the operative field. Local myocardial cooling is another useful adjunct accomplished simply by dripping saline through small intravenous tubing directly onto a small gauze square on the heart so that the fluid spreads diffusely over the surface of the heart into the pericardial sac. A small suction tube situated near the cardiac incision prevents the pericardial bath fluid spilling into the heart. We feel this has been particularly useful in infants with complex forms of transposition of the great arteries or complete AV canal, where the period of circulatory arrest or myocardial ischemia tends to be over 45 min in length, thus placing the myocardium in jeopardy if it was to rewarm.

To indicate more of the problems and indications, our clinical experience is reviewed briefly.

Clinical Experience

Over the total period, 516 of 689 patients (75%) survived (fig.1). There has been a steady improvement in survival with increased experience in both the application of hypothermia and the technical repair of the various defects. Over the last 21 months, 156 of 189 (83%) survived. Further improvement should be expected. For instance, an analysis of our cases revealed a number in whom the period of circulatory arrest was prolonged relative to the degree of hypothermia. Circulatory arrest or ischemic myocardial arrest at 20°C should be limited to 45 min. Prolonged ischemia causes myocardial damage and low cardiac output. Where a complicated repair requires more time, this can be obtained either by cooling to a lower temperature, or by completing a portion of the repair on cardiopulmonary bypass or low-flow

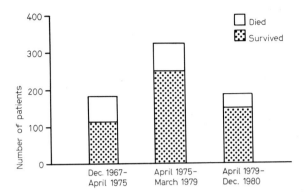

Fig. 1. From 1967 to December 1980, 516 of 689 patients (75%) survived. There has been a steady improvement with 83% surviving in the most recent time period.

bypass. Combining a limited period of circulatory arrest with a period of low or normal flow cardiopulmonary bypass when repairing complicated defects has reduced the incidence of low output cardiac failure and has increased survival.

The mortality rate for the entire series was also related to several other aspects of patient distribution. In general, the mortality rate was higher in patients under 6 months of age than in those over 6 months of age. Similarly, the mortality rate was greater in infants under 5 kg body weight compared to infants over 5 kg. Later in the series, these factors were less important. As one would expect, children with conditions considered urgent or semi-urgent had a higher mortality than children operated on electively. Significant early postoperative complications, such as myocardial failure and pulmonary atelectasis were frequent. It has been suggested that these problems are less common with surface cooling since core cooling is associated with more capillary leak and metabolic problems, but we have no significant comparable data.

The series may be further distributed according to the specific type of cardiovascular defect. In general, the mortality rate was highest among patients with the more complex less frequently encountered lesions, and where only palliative or incomplete repairs could be accomplished. Patients chosen for repair with deep hypothermia and circulatory arrest rather than with standard cardiopulmonary bypass were generally under 10 kg body weight and less than 2 years of age.

Ventricular Septal Defect

There were 32 deaths in 205 patients. Recent mortality rate is 10%. Closure of the ventricular septal defect was routinely accomplished by the transatrial route. 75% of the patients who died had either multiple ventricular septal defects (VSD) or associated intracardiac lesions. Only 25% of the survivors had associated cardiac lesions.

Since most repairs can be completed in 30–40 min, hypothermia and circulatory arrest is an appropriate method of managing VSD in infancy, and for the most part should avoid the need for palliative pulmonary artery banding. There is a limited place for pulmonary artery banding however, particularly in small infants who are very sick or with complicated muscular or multiple ventricular septal defects. The presence of an associated malformation may or may not be an indication for a palliative procedure, for it may be preferable to attempt repair of both defects. We note that some surgeons are using other techniques in infancy, but it is not clear why one should not use deep hypothermia.

Transposition of the Great Arteries

168 patients with transposition of the great arteries (TGA) underwent intra-atrial repair. There were 18 deaths. Most patients who died had complex transposition of great arteries with either associated VSD or pulmonary stenosis or both. There were 3 deaths in the infants with transposition and intact ventricular septum, all early in the series.

The use of deep hypothermia and circulatory arrest has simplified the repair of TGA in infants. It is particularly useful in uncomplicated transposition because the repair can be carried out within the safe limits afforded by cooling to a rectal temperature of 18 °C or below. When there is an associated VSD or pulmonary stenosis, the safe time may be exceeded, thus increasing postoperative morbidity and mortality. This should be avoided by carefully limiting the period of myocardial ischemia, doing part of the repair on cardiopulmonary bypass with good myocardial perfusion or, possibly as an alternative, cooling to a lower temperature. Selecting some infants for arterial repair should reduce mortality.

Total Anomalous Pulmonary Venous Drainage

76 patients underwent repair of total anomalous pulmonary venous drainage with 22 deaths (29%). Recent mortality is 6%. The majority of patients were repaired in the first 4 months of life. The best results were in the infants with infra-diaphragmatic drainage.

Hypothermia with circulatory arrest remains the most favorable approach to these infants. The mortality rate has improved in recent years chiefly due to earlier operation and improved postoperative care.

Complete AV Canal

There were 79 patients in this group with 30 deaths (38 %). Recent mortality is 25 %. Of those who died, many had associated anomalies, e. g. hypoplastic mitral valve, multiple VSD, hypoplastic right ventricle with infundibular stenosis and parachute mitral valve which ideally should be diagnosed preoperatively and palliated. Myocardial failure from prolonged ischemia, breakdown of the valve repair and sepsis were important causes of death and indicate the need for careful technique and management. Most infants require repair before the age of 24 months, either to control cardiac failure or prevent pulmonary vascular disease. Pulmonary artery banding is reserved for children with difficult complex problems, such as multiple muscular VSD, hypoplastic right ventricle, etc.

Deep hypothermia and circulatory arrest is ideal for repair of the AV canal except that the repair may take more time than is afforded by a single episode of circulatory arrest. Cooling to lower temperatures or doing the last part of the repair on cardiopulmonary bypass is necessary to avoid this problem. Many of these infants are in chronic heart failure before operation and the myocardium does not have the reserve to tolerate a long period of ischemia. Low-flow hypothermic bypass is a useful adjunct in some of these cases.

Pulmonary Atresia or Stenosis

This is a diverse group of patients. 15 of the patients had pulmonary stenosis with intact septum and there were 2 deaths in this group. 11 patients had pulmonary atresia with intact septum. 6 patients died. There were 3 patients who had pulmonary atresia with VSD; 1 survived right ventricular outflow tract reconstruction, leaving the VSD open. Although deep hypothermic circulatory arrest is a convenient method of managing these lesions, often they are more simply repaired on low-flow bypass.

Tetralogy of Fallot

19 of 26 patients survived repair of tetralogy of Fallot among a varied group of infants which included cases with absent pulmonary valve, anomalous left coronary artery, critical aortic stenosis and complete AV canal. Generally, we prefer to shunt infants in the first 2 years of life. After the age of 2, tetralogy of Fallot is repaired, but with cardiopulmonary bypass. In

infancy, deep hypothermia and circulatory arrest can be used for tetralogy repair, but other techniques, such as low-flow or standard bypass, are equally effective and likely safer.

Deep hypothermia and circulatory arrest is a convenient way of managing certain other congenital cardiac malformations in infancy, such as interrupted aortic arch, atrial septal defect and some cases of double outlet right ventricle. Some other conditions, such as aortic stenosis and truncus arteriosus are better managed on bypass with low-flow. In the case of truncus arteriosus, the management plan employed by *Ebert* seems ideal with a combination of short periods of aortic cross-clamping and hypothermic low-flow bypass. It is likely that the infant with truncus arteriosus and high run-off from systemic to pulmonary circulations has poor myocardial perfusion before operation. Thus, this infant has little tolerance for myocardial ischemia and any interruption in aortic perfusion must be short. To some extent, the same must hold true for sick infants with complete AV canal and VSD.

There are a number of miscellaneous complex malformations which required tailored surgical management and are usually associated with a high risk. Frequently, the profound hypothermia and circulatory arrest technique is very convenient for identifying and treating these problems.

Of common concern is the question of cerebral damage from the period of circulatory arrest. Early in the series, we had 12 children with residual neurologic defects, mostly minor and temporary as a result of exceeding the safe limit allowed by the temperature to which the child had been cooled. In a separate review, *Steward* [10] at the Hospital for Sick Children, Toronto, reviewed the first 400 consecutive patients undergoing profound hypothermia and circulatory arrest. He found that there were 276 early and 262 late survivors in this group. Of these 262 patients, 14 had had significant neurologic sequelae. But of these 14 patients, 13 of them had some peri-operative event other than circulatory arrest which may have caused the neurologic deficit. Only patient 14 had no associated event to explain his deficit. Further, *Haka-Ikse* et al. [4] in a detailed review of 17 randomly selected patients who had undergone profound hypothermia and circulatory arrest found no significant impairment of psychomotor ability in these patients when compared with other children with similar cardiac defects.

The results with profound hypothermia and circulatory arrest continue to improve. The mortality in the last 2 years has been 17%. It continues to be a useful technique which provides excellent exposure for accurate repair of major and complex cardiac defects in infants.

References

1   Bailey, L.L.; Takeuchi, Y.; Williams, W.G.; Trusler, G.A.; Mustard, W.T.: Surgical management of congenital cardiovascular anomalies with the use of profound hypothermia and circulatory arrest; analysis of 180 cases. J.thorac.cardiovasc.Surg. *71:* 485 (1976).

2   Barrett-Boyes, B.G.; Simpson, M.; Neutze, J.M.: Intracardiac surgery in neonates and infants using deep hypothermia with surface cooling and limited cardiopulmonary bypass. Circulation *43:* 1–25 (1971).

3   Ebert, P.A.; Robinson, S.J.; Stanger, P.; Engle, M.A.: Pulmonary artery conduits in infants younger than six months of age. J.thorac.cardiovasc.Surg. *72:* 3, 351 (1976).

4   Haka-Ikse, K.; Blackwood, M.J.; Steward, D.J.: Psychomotor development of infants and children after profound hypothermia during surgery for congenital heart disease. Devl.Med.Child Neur. *20:* 62–70 (1978).

5   Horiuchi, T.; Koyamada, K.; Matano, I.; et al.: Radical operation for ventricular septal defect in infancy. J.thorac.cardiovasc.Surg. *46:* 180–190 (1963).

6   Johnson, A.E.; Radde, I.C.; Steward, D.J.; Taylor, J.: Acid-base and electrolyte changes in infants undergoing profound hypothermia for surgical correction of congenital heart defects. Can.Anaesth.Soc.J. *21:* 23–45 (1974).

7   Mohri, H.; Dillard, D.H.; Crawford, E.W.; Martin, W.E.; Merendino, K.A.: Method of surface induced deep hypothermia for open-heart surgery in infants J.thorac.Surg. *58:* 262–270 (1969).

8   Muraoka, R.; Hikasa, Y.; Shirotani, I.I. et al.: Open-heart surgery in infants under two years of age using deep hypothermia with surface cooling and partial cardiopulmonary bypass. J.cardiovasc.Surg. *15:* 231–241 (1974).

9   Roe, R.B.; Hutchinson, J.C.; Fishman, N.H.; Ullyot, D.J.; Smith, D.L.: Myocardial protection with cold, ischemic, potassium-induced cardioplegia. J.thorac.cardiovasc.Surg. *73:* 366 (1977).

10 Steward, D.J.: Anesthesia for complex congenital anomalies. Cleveland Clin.Q. *48:* 166 (1981).

George A.Trusler, Associate Professor of Surgery, University of Toronto, School of Medicine, Head, Division of Cardiovascular Surgery, The Hospital for Sick Children, Toronto, Ont. (Canada)

Mod. Probl. Paediat., vol. 22, pp. 210–215 (Karger, Basel 1983)

Postoperative Monitoring of Pediatric Cardiac Patients

Gordon K. Danielson

Department of Surgery, Mayo Foundation, Mayo Clinic, Mayo Graduate School of Medicine, Rochester, Minn., USA

This will be a brief review of the current monitoring practices of the cardiac surgeons at the Mayo Clinic where over 1,200 open-heart procedures are performed each year, approximately 350 of which are for congenital heart disease. In addition to the usual nursing monitoring of temperature, pulse, respiration, and intake and output, a number of other variables are monitored. These are perhaps best classified according to subsystems.

Table I shows the monitoring for the cardiac subsystem. Oscilloscopic electrocardiography is essential. Its usefulness is enhanced firstly by the availability of a memory loop or scope hold that retains 4–10 s of electrocardiographic rhythm, and secondly by a direct writing capability that gives an on-line electrocardiogram or reproduces the stored rhythm. An arrhythmia alarm can be combined with the electrocardiogram which is triggered by either asystole, bradyarrhythmias, tachyarrhythmias, or ventricular fibrillation. This is best done by a computer system which will be described subsequently.

We monitor routinely left atrial pressure in all patients who have a left atrial vent inserted at the time of operation. Right atrial pressure is also monitored on all patients by inserting a catheter into the right atrial appendage following removal of the venous cannulae. A Sorenson flush system is employed to keep the catheters free of clots (Intraflow continuous flush system, No. CFS–O3F, Sorenson Research Co., Salt Lake City, Utah).

Arterial pressure is also monitored in all complicated cases with an indwelling Teflon catheter (Longdwel Teflon catheter-needle, Becton-Dickinson and Co., Rutherford, N.J.). The catheter can be inserted percutaneously in most adults and older children.

Very useful indirect measures of cardiac output are the right atrial pO_2

Table I. Cardiac monitoring

1	Oscilloscopic electrocardiography
	(a) Memory loop and direct writing capability
	(b) Arrhythmia alarm
2	Left atrial pressure
3	Right atrial pressure
4	Arterial pressures (systolic, diastolic, pulse)
5	Right atrial pO_2 and saturation
6	Arterial pO_2 and saturation
7	Extremity color, temperature, pulses, capillary filling
8	Cardiac output
	(a) Dye curves
	(b) Thermodilution
	(c) Pulse pressure methods
9	Blood volume

and saturation. If the patient's hemoglobin, temperature, and level of activity remain relatively stable, the right atrial saturations and pO_2 are a good reflection of the adequacy of cardiac output. Levels above 50–60 % saturation are compatible with satisfactory cardiac outout. Trends in the saturation are particularly useful; a falling saturation may be the first clue to a deteriorating cardiac output.

Some indication of cardiac output can be derived from noting the color, temperature, pulses and capillary filling of the patient's extremities. One can run the back of one's hand down the patient's leg towards the feet and notice the level where the extremity becomes colder. Evaluation of effectiveness of various interventions can be quickly determined by noting whether the level of coldness moves further towards the toes. We have not routinely monitored extremity temperature and compared it with core temperature, but others have found this temperature gradient to be a sensitive indicator of adequacy of perfusion.

Cardiac output can be determined by direct measurement. The dye method is limited by the quantity of blood required for calibration and for performance of the circulation curves. We have not found the dye method completely suitable for infants and young children. The thermodilution technique offers a relatively simple method for repeated determinations without significant blood loss, but precise attention to details is important for reproducible results. Pulse pressure methods in our hands have not been reliable because the changing peripheral resistance of postoperative patients invalidates the calibration curves.

We have not found blood volume determinations to be very useful in the immediate postoperative period. Blood volumes are of some help in the first postoperative day when hemodynamics have stabilized and chest drainage is minimal. Occasionally, one is surprised to find that the blood volume is significantly greater or significantly less than was suspected clinically.

Table II shows the monitoring for the pulmonary subsystem. Determinations of arterial pH, pO_2, saturation and pCO_2 are made on all patients at least twice on the night following operation. For patients on ventilators and others who are not doing well, more frequent blood gas determinations are made. Monitoring of the inflation pressure for patients on ventilators is useful in following the effective compliance and is a guide to help with the decision concerning extubation. Tidal volume, respiratory frequency, and minute volume are recorded by the respiratory therapy team at frequent intervals, and are adjusted as necessary according to the blood gas values. Some respirators now have small computers which allow calculation of airway resistance, lung compliance, functional residual capacity, and other respiratory variables; these are helpful for evaluating patients with difficult cardiopulmonary problems, particularly with regard to consideration of extubation, but are not used routinely.

Insertion of a urinary catheter is not necessary or routine unless the patient has had a long, complex operation or is developing signs of a low cardiac output postoperatively. For adults, we like to keep the urine output greater than 20 ml/h and, for infants less than 1 year, greater than 1 ml/kg/h. A fall in urine output is an early sign of cardiac tamponade and also of low cardiac output. One of the variables to watch during therapeutic intervention for low cardiac output is an improvement in urinary output. Measurement of urine osmolality is occasionally helpful in managing patients, particularly for detecting dehydration in infants (greater than 300 mosm/l).

Finally, metabolic monitoring is important, particularly in infants less than 1 year old. Hypocalcemia and hypoglycemia can occur quickly in infants, so frequent determinations of serum calcium and blood sugar are performed in the first 24 h postoperatively. Serum electrolytes and creatinine levels are measured at appropriate intervals in all patients. As the serum potassium can change quickly, particularly in the presence of vigorous diuresis or renal insufficiency, serum levels are obtained several times during the first postoperative night.

In summary, one probably does not need to monitor anything other than vital signs in the majority of patients who will do well without any special intervention. For the infant, for those who undergo long operations

Table II. Pulmonary monitoring

1	Arterial pH, pO_2, saturation, pCO_2
2	Inflation pressure, end-expiratory pressure
3	Tidal volume, respiratory frequency, minute volume
4	Airway resistance, lung compliance, functional residual capacity

for complex congenital cardiac defects, and for those patients with significant impairment of myocardial function, proper and complete monitoring is essential for a successful outcome.

In a cooperative effort between International Business Machines and the Mayo Clinic, a venture in computer-based intensive care monitoring was initiated in January 1972. The basic monitoring system can be divided into three subsets [1]. The first is a bedside monitoring cart with built-in preprocessors for temperature, chest drainage, urine output, and pressure measurements. The purposes of the preprocessors are: (1) to reduce the amount of central computer sampling, and (2) to provide direct digital values of mean systolic and diastolic pressures for the three hemodynamic catheters.

The second subset is an on-site dedicated System 7 IBM computer with 32K memory capability and the third subset is a central 'parent' 370–135 IBM computer which is used for back-up and data analysis.

Computer keyboards for entering and recalling data are located at the bedside and are designed for optimal computer interaction with personnel. A color-coded keyboard emphasizes the several types of computer interaction. Red keys provide access to patient files for entering or erasing data. Conversely, green keys indicate 'safe' computer use and encourage review of stored data. Special function keys labeled 'hemodynamic display', 'blood balance', 'fluid balance', 'laboratory data', and the like provide immediate access to those displays most frequently reviewed.

Left and right atrial pressures, chest and urine drainage, and respiratory rate (Monaghan) are sampled and displayed every 2 min. If the measured values in this sampling are beyond preset deviations of the previous recordings, two additional samples are obtained at 20-second intervals to determine whether the reading in question was a temporary fluctuation or a true value. The blood pressure values are based on the mean value of 10 consecutive beat analyses with elimination of the highest and lowest readings. The most recent data sample to pass the validity check is then displayed numerically at the end of a line graph, which plots the variable in real time sequence. In

Table III. Computerized versus standard cardiac intensive care unit

	Intensive care unit, patients (%)	
Factors	computerized: 450 patients	standard: 378 patients
Duration of stay, days	2.6	2.6
Vasopressor support	74 (16)	59 (16)
Antiarrhythmic drugs	117 (26)	69 (18)
Serious arrhythmias	35 (8)	29 (8)
Mortality	11 (2)	13 (3)
Arrhythmia-related death	4 (1)	10 (3)

contrast to the 2-min sampling interval for these relatively stable variables, the electrocardiogram is continuously sampled and analysed on an individual beat-to-beat basis.

A system of computer logic was developed to aid recognition of potential problems. A message light could be activated if any of a number of variables exceeded set limits. For example, an arterial systolic pressure less than 70 mm Hg, an increase in chest drainage in a 15-min interval of 75 ml or more over the average of the two previous 15-min intervals, or electrocardiographic abnormalities were programmed to light a message light. Also available is a catastrophe logic based on pulse recognition correlated with the electrocardiogram which provides for recognition of various serious rhythm disturbances and for differentiation of artifacts.

The computer has also been programmed to provide for infusion of blood or drugs according to preset limits for left atrial pressure, blood pressure, chest tube drainage, and heart rate. Further evaluations of other applications are planned.

A 6-month comparative study was made between a computerized cardiac intensive care unit (12 beds) and another unit which has full monitoring services without computer linkage (10 beds). Patients were randomly assigned before operation to one or the other units. The assignment was made within three categories: (1) open or closed surgical procedure, (2) emergency or elective surgery, and (3) age of patient. Nursing personnel were rotated between the two units to avoid bias.

Distribution of the categories of the 828 patients between the units was similar, although the numbers were somewhat greater in the larger unit (table III). There was no significant difference in duration of stay between the two units. A similar percentage of patients in each unit needed vaso-pressor support. There was a greater use of anti-arrhythmic drugs in the com-puterized unit (p < 0.01); this may have been due to an increased awareness of arrhythmias by the nursing and medical personnel in the computerized unit. The number of serious arrhythmias, however, was the same in both units. The mortality was slightly higher in the standard unit, but this difference was not statistically significant. Thus, while the computer facilitates some aspects of postoperative care, it is difficult to show that it favorably affects mortality or morbidity. Of far greater importance is the constant presence of trained staff, including a member of the cardiac surgical team.

Reference

1   Danielson, G.K.; Pluth, J.R.; Smith, H.C.; Schultz, G.L.: Postoperative monitor-ing at the Mayo Clinic; in Anderson, Shinebourne, Paediatric cardiology, 1977, chap.9, pp.70–75 (Churchill-Livingstone, Edinburgh 1978).

Gordon K.Danielson, MD, Department of Surgery, Mayo Foundation, Mayo Clinic, Mayo Graduate School of Medicine, Rochester, MN 55905 (USA)

MAY CIRCULATE FOR 2 WEEKS